HOSPITAL SECURITY AND SAFETY

A. Michael Pascal

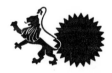

ASPEN SYSTEMS CORPORATION
GERMANTOWN, MARYLAND
1977

RA969.95
P37

Library of Congress Cataloging in Publication Data

Pascal, A. Michael.
Hospital security and safety.

Includes index.
1. Hospitals — Security measures.
2. Hospitals — Safety measures. I. Title.
RA969.95.P37   658.47   77-14083
ISBN 0-89443-029-7

Library of Congress Catalog Card Number: 77-14083
ISBN: 0-89443-029-7

Printed in the United States of America

1 2 3 4 5

*To Harry and Bernie, without whom
this book would not have been possible.*

Table of Contents

Foreword

A patient, visitor, or physician stepping into a hospital needs to believe that the institution is a haven of safety, healing, rest, and security from the pressures of the outside world. Invariably, the physician feels a sense of warmth. Here is a secure place where one may practice the healing arts without the effects of the adverse influences too often accepted as commonplace in the outside world.

But in reality, these institutions are staffed by people possessing all of the frailties found in the outside world. Unfortunately, real people mean real problems. Emergency situations and thefts requiring the control of an effective security force are prevalent.

To the physician and the hospital administrator, this is a concise, direct, forthright book that presents the problems and the solutions in a logical and clear sequence — just how security should *and can* work in a hospital.

Michael Pascal has not been frivolous in his approach. This book is a logical mixture of necessary realism and Yankee conservatism. The theme is constantly that of getting the highest quality results for the best spent dollars. And Mr. Pascal's experience in all aspects of the hospital security field is evident throughout.

For those of us who are conditioned not to think about hospitals as security problems, *Hospital Security and Safety* is a mandatory eye-opener. For administrators plagued by spiraling costs, this volume should be required reading, and the security methods recommended required applications.

I feel confident that the careful reading of *Hospital Security and Safety* and the employment of the concepts presented would doubtlessly mean cost-effective security for any medical facility, regardless of size.

John W. Heisse, Jr., M.D.

Preface

The day when hospital security was defined as merely a guard making rounds in the medical area has certainly gone by. Today, more sophisticated programs are needed to ensure the day-to-day safety and security of the staff, employees, patients, and visitors.

My aim in this book is to present the basic requirements for effective facility security, and the methods for fulfilling those requirements, in such a manner that any responsible hospital administrator can effectively begin and control an efficient system of protection and prevention. Then, as the facility grows, so too must security. When facility growth reaches the preordained expectancy ceiling, the administrator can *and should* turn the existing security system prototype over to a professional and capable security director.

Too many publications that present this type of information outline, assume, and, in fact, strongly advise a close tie between law-enforcement techniques and facility security. I have taken an almost completely different turn; *civil* law rather than *criminal* law is the foundation of my approach. I do not intend to imply that the principles of criminal law do not have some potential application in facility security matters. What I do emphasize, however, is that such application must only be "kept in mind" while we concentrate on the application of the principles and techniques of civil law, which, with common sense and firmly established security controls, shall allow the hospital administrator and/or the security director to respond to any and all situations. Use of outside agency personnel heavily schooled in criminal law techniques may not be necessary; a fully trained in-house staff and the application of enforced controls will prove infinitely more cost-effective.

Why and how any responsible hospital administrator can justify a cutback of security expenditures as a savings is completely beyond my comprehension. It represents one of the greatest business fallacies of all time; it represents *reaction* instead of *action*. When a budget cut appears necessary, the responsible administrator will call in the security director and request a report as to where, in fact, security dollars, in any form, are being wasted. The security director, if a professional, will have such information readily available as a result of the routine reports received from the security staff. After thorough analysis and consultation with the security director, the administrator might find areas that could be reasonably cut. It remains imperative, however, that the administrator clearly realize that a severe cutback or cancellation of security only opens the door to theft and uncontrolled emergencies that can represent infinitely greater costs than the security expenditure that was supposedly saved. Nothing could be as costly as inefficient security.

A. Micheal Pascal

Acknowledgments

I deeply thank the many friends, acquaintances, and business associates who gave me the experience and knowledge to write a book on a much-needed subject—medical facility security. The names of those who gave much time, thought, and information to this project are listed below.

Joseph Austin, Jr., Massachusetts Hospital Association, Burlington, Massachusetts
David Balesi, McClean Hospital, Belmont, Massachusetts
Donna M. Calcagno, Braintree, Massachusetts
Thomas Hannon, Springfield, Massachusetts
Dr. John W. Heisse, Jr., Burlington, Vermont
John P. Henebry, Jr., Pacific Inspections, Los Angeles, California
John King, Springfield, Massachusetts
Edmund J. Kinter, Leonard Morse Hospital, Natick Massachusetts
Dean Timothy Moran, Northeastern University, Boston, Massachusetts
Victor J. Piscitello, Victor Service Bureau, Lawrence, Massachusetts
Ernest C. Reid, Boston, Massachusetts

Additionally, I have gained invaluable knowledge and experience by serving as consultant for, or by establishing the security programs of the following institutions, and am extremely grateful.

Beth Israel Hospital, Boston, Massachusetts
Boston Hospital for Women, Boston, Massachusetts
Peter Bent Brigham Hospital, Boston, Massachusetts
Robert B. Brigham Hospital, Roxbury, Massachusetts
Brookline Hospital, Brookline, Massachusetts
Cambridge Hospital, Cambridge, Massachusetts

Children's Hospital, Los Angeles, California
Children's Hospital Medical Center, Roxbury, Massachusetts
Framingham Union Hospital, Framingham, Massachusetts
Glover Memorial Hospital, Needham, Massachusetts
Grover Manor Hospital, Revere, Massachusetts
Hebrew Rehabilitation Center for the Aged, Roslindale, Massachusetts
Jimmy Fund Cancer Research Facility, Boston, Massachusetts
Joslin Clinic, Boston, Massachusetts
Kennedy Memorial Hospital for Children, Brighton, Massachusetts
Lahey Clinic Foundation, Boston, Massachusetts
Lynn Hospital, Lynn, Massachusetts
Lynn Union Hospital, Lynn, Massachusetts
Massachusetts College of Pharmacy, Boston, Massachusetts
Massachusetts Hospital Association, Burlington, Massachusetts
Mattapan Chronic Disease Hospital, Cambridge, Massachusetts
McLean Hospital, Belmont, Massachusetts
Melrose-Wakefield Hospital, Melrose, Massachusetts
Leonard Morse Hospital, Natick, Massachusetts
New England Deaconess Hospital, Boston, Massachusetts
Newton-Wellesley Hospital, Newton, Massachusetts
Sacred Heart Hospital, Manchester, New Hampshire
St. Elizabeth's Hospital, Brighton, Massachusetts
St. John of God Hospital, Brighton, Massachusetts
St. Margaret's Hospital for Women, Dorchester, Massachusetts
Simmons College, Boston, Massachusetts
Somerville Hospital, Somerville, Massachusetts
Waltham Hospital, Waltham, Massachusetts
Wiswall Hospital, Wellesley, Massachusetts

Youville Rehabilitation and Chronic Disease Hospital, Cambridge,
Massachusetts

Part I
Organizational Requirements

Chapter 1

Identification of Needs And Priorities

How can you create a more efficient, cost-effective security system utilizing current personnel and equipment to greatest advantage and enlarging areas where existing coverage is lacking? Essentially, to begin to organize your priorities, you have to learn exactly what your needs are and become knowledgeable about the various alternatives available for meeting those needs. Questions you must begin to answer are:

1. Does your facility require a new inhouse security force or an outside agency staff, or is it necessary only to expand or refine your present system?
2. How can particularly vulnerable areas be made effectively secure?
3. How can day-to-day performance standards of your security force be improved?
4. Are physical changes to your facility necessary?
5. How can you effectively combine security personnel and mechanical/electronic surveillance equipment?

DEPARTMENTAL INPUT

The most efficient first step in determining your security needs is an organized study of existing security coverage, with input from all department heads regarding constructive changes and/or expansions within the system. Hold meetings with your department heads, at which each departmental security need is presented, recorded, and discussed. The record of the meetings, listing existing problems and all suggestions for solutions, should be transcribed along with a detailed summary of the existing security system.

THE PROFESSIONAL CONSULTANT

Once you have defined existing problems and detailed the existing system, you should hire a professional security consultant to draft proposals concerning structure and budgetary allotments of the new security system.

Initially, you should contact more than one professional consultant. Check references and professional background to assure that the consultant you ultimately hire is indeed a recognized authority. Once you have hired a consultant, follow that consultant's advice.

The final specifications of your security system shall, of course, be designed by the consultant, who should, among other things, insist that part of the security system be composed of qualified investigators to supervise personnel of security officer status. Also, the consultant should set up your reporting procedure so that one copy of every report dealing with the security functions for the week goes to the chief executive officer of the facility. Copies of your security reports should also reach each member of the board of directors of the facility so that every aspect of the security function is known to everyone involved in facility management. These are just two examples of the comprehensiveness that should pervade all aspects of your consultant's plan; specific steps will be discussed in detail in the following chapters. The importance of mentioning it here should be clear—you have to be wary of the "professional" consultant who takes what could prove to be expensive shortcuts.

INHOUSE STAFF VS. OUTSIDE AGENCY

In the event that the facility involved does not appear large enough to support its own inhouse security director, investigators, and security staff, the consultant should make provisions to hire a professional outside agency to furnish qualified personnel. Under no circumstances should one mix an outside agency with inhouse security employees. The obvious exception to this general rule is the use of an individual outside consultant, as discussed.

The facility administrator who considers the use of an outside agency must be wary of the promises of agency sales representatives. When an unwary administrator signs a contract for the services of an agency, and both parties are positive that they are in complete accord with each other, trouble may still be brewing. The administrator returns to more demanding responsibilities and awaits fulfillment of the contract. When the sales representative returns to the agency office with the signed contract, agency management may interpret the purposely vague clauses in the contract differently, to fit the actual capabilities of the agency. As a result, the client facility may or may not get the amount or quality of security personnel contracted. I can fairly well guarantee that the operation and administration of the terms of the contract will in no way represent the discussion held prior to the signing of the contract.

To guard against this situation, the facility administrator is well advised to ensure that all aspects of the agency hiring are witnessed by the facility's staff assistants and/or attorneys. Any and all reports submitted by the agency must be addressed to only one individual at the client facility, with copies to the individual's supervisor. The contract and subsequent operations must be dictated by the administrator of the facility directly to the on-premises senior representative of the agency. It must be clearly understood that no one but the facility administrator has the authority to change in any way the orders affecting the on-premises operation of the agency. The agency management must be completely prohibited from issuing to any of their subordinates any type of orders concerning the facility operation. The contract must specifically state that violations of this and all other safeguarding clauses in the contract nulls the contract. In other words, the facility uses the agency not as a security or personnel policy-determining agency, but rather as an *employment* service. The actual application of the security personnel will be directed and dictated by the client facility administrator through the inhouse security director, and definitively specified in the contract.

As further guarantee that the contracted agency will indeed provide the services needed, the facility administrator must demand an ironclad guarantee that all "special agents," guards, etc. shall be well and truly trained and thus completely capable of doing the job properly. Being guaranteed verbally by the sales representative obviously does not suffice; it must appear in writing. And the administrator must further insist that a "training clause" fully explain what "training" shall mean—how comprehensive it is, who conducts it, and what determines its successful completion by the individual trainee. As an overall check on quality, investigate the personnel hiring criteria of the contracted agency. Equally important, the administrator must be totally satisfied that the agency's on-premises senior representative has additional training, effective leadership qualities, and a cooperative attitude regarding facility management. Be generally cautious, obviously, when dealing with an ego-inflated "chief special agent." Regarding all agency personnel, your insistence must be on *quality*, and the definition of "quality" must be determined and mandated by the facility administrator, not the agency.

MANNED SECURITY POSTS VS. ELECTRONIC COVERAGE

Regardless of which type of security personnel you finally decide to use, you must ensure that all areas mandating security are in fact covered. You must establish where and when stationary security is required, and how many people are needed. You must do the same with any roving patrols that may be required. As you go about setting up these posts or stations, and their staffing and equipment requirements, you must continually review all that occurs within the building and grounds (traffic flow, hours of concentrated activity, etc.), and then assign posts so that you get the most return on your security expenditure.

In the type of facilities with which we are dealing, a "post" would range from a single stationary and a single roving patrol to any number of each that is required. Here the key word is *required*; at no time should a security post be established unless it shall, by its very existence, be cost-effective. To place a guard at a door merely because the door leads to the exterior or to a specialized area can become a great waste of both money and personnel. There are certainly security stations that absolutely demand human coverage; but mechanized and/or electronic equipment can effectively replace guards at several posts. For example, areas that are completely closed off during nonduty hours can be sufficiently covered by locks and alarms. There is actually no reason to add human coverage, although an agency might suggest such personnel use for "firewatch" purposes. I would consider such advice questionable. A roving patrol could indeed discover a fire; but just as certainly, so could an alarm system, which would cost less, automatically alert centralized personnel at the stationary post, and proceed to act upon the fire with automatic sprinklers while the stationary personnel proceeded to call for further assistance. Surveillance by the added person at the scene is neither efficient nor cost-effective. The money could be better utilized in installing and maintaining mechanical and/or electronic devices *keyed in* to a centralized manned station.

In dollars and cents, I am talking of a savings of many thousands of dollars per year. At today's wages, $2.75 to $3.50 per hour, in one year of 313 eight-hour shifts from midnight to 8:00 a.m. (2,504 hours), a roving "firewatch" would cost $6,886 ($2.75/hour) to $8,764 ($3.50/hour). In this same year, you have at least 52 24-hour shifts (1,248 hours) for Sunday coverage, at the rate of at least time and a half; you also have approximately eight paid holidays at double time. Therefore, add at least another $5,154 per person for Sunday coverage and approximately $1,056 for paid holidays. In total, you are paying at least $13,076 per year per person. And the cost increases on a yearly basis. In addition to this expenditure, you have probably already expended at least a similar amount for protection via the installed automatic sprinkler system that works whether your guard is there or not. To emphasize: I recently reviewed the security expenditure of a large retail chain and was able to cut their yearly expenditure from $247,170 to $216,964 — while simultaneously improving their security by substituting mechanical/electronic *protection* for human *coverage*.

Therefore, it makes more sense to install efficient burglar and fire-alarm response systems, which have relatively small annual maintenance fees, than to pay out money for guards who cannot match the efficiency of automatic systems. Naturally, an agency interested in providing you with personnel will lean toward personnel as a solution to all security problems. You must carefully review your needs and expand surveillance with devices when it becomes obvious that by so doing you can cut down expenditures while increasing protection.

There are many additional ways in which mechanical and/or electronic coverage can save money. For example, it can expand personnel security and monitor personnel arrival and departure for payroll reasons as well as inhouse security. With a single stationary security post at your employees' entrance serving as the central nerve center, other points of building entrance can be closed off, with entry being gained only through security clearance via audio and video control from the nerve center. Access to the building is then completely covered. More savings can be realized by adding an employee ID card to your payroll functions. Each employee would then be required to show the ID card in order to gain access to the facility. The card could be coded to allow either full or limited access. And upon reporting to work, the employee would insert the card in a special lock or device that would verify the card and record the date and time of arrival. The entry record would thereby also function as a payroll record for the cardholder, thus eliminating the need for separate time clocks and time cards.

Summary

Major steps and decisions to be made at the outset of your attempts to establish or refine a facility-wide security system include: a staff-oriented discussion of needs, including an outline of the existing security system and its obvious shortcomings; consideration and hiring of an acceptable professional security consultant; careful consideration concerning the formulation of your own inhouse security staff or the contracting of an outside agency; and the possible substitution of mechanical and/or electronic devices for a burgeoning force of unneeded and costly security guards.

Chapter 2

The Professional Survey

As discussed in Chapter 1, determining the facility's security needs must begin with input from all facility department heads. As I have recommended, the professional consultant should then be called in. Equipped with the information gathered from departmental staff and the resultant outline of the existing system and its obvious shortcomings, the professional consultant will conduct an overall survey designed to advise you concerning the precise amount of security you need and the most cost-effective and efficient methods available. This professional survey should give you a complete working outline, including the comparative costs of an outside agency vs. the inhouse staff. The outline should indicate both minimum standards and maximum need; your final security system can then be built, taking into consideration both need and financial ability. The professional survey should represent a comprehensive, overall plan; new features should not merely be tacked on to the existing system. The result should be the proper amount and kind of coverage.

Here again, the administrator must be cautious, and should demand that the survey be all-inclusive. To help you ensure an acceptable survey, I will outline a checklist of items that must be covered.

Perimeter

The survey must include a comprehensive description and analysis of the area in which the facility is located. Such information should include a complete listing of: the social, economic, and crime-rate history of the area; the present crime-rate standing, including fire and police protection, and how it could affect you; population and zoning trends in the area; and traffic flow on all surrounding roads, including capacity, routing, and general patterns. The natural property boundaries of the facility and existing man-made boundaries, such as fences, should be analyzed, as should all existing exterior lighting systems and protective alarms. Based on the hospital location, the survey should also attempt to forecast the socioeconomic portrait of potential employees, patients, and neighboring residents and businesspeople. This portrait may prove valuable in determining whether extra security might be necessary for demonstrations, vandalism, etc.

The survey should also provide the administrator with specific recommendations concerning necessary *physical security* (locks, doors, barriers, etc.) and *controls* (keys, documents, personnel, vehicles, merchandise movement, etc.). An effective system of properly administered controls can save you the yearly cost of your security department. This has been proven time and time again. Conversely, you can lose double or triple the cost of your security department if the systems are not properly administered. In Chapter 3 I will cover some basic systems of controls.

Parking Lots

The parking facility portion of the survey should include recommended placement of lot and most efficient placement of cars within the lot. A major question to be answered by the consultant is whether the lot security will be manned or mechanized. Parking security for employees should also include a pass and registration system for users. This aspect of security control is perhaps the least understood and most certainly the least appreciated, yet it ranks as one of the more valuable jobs performed by the security department. It is essential that the problems in this area of the facility's operation be presented properly, and that facility management cooperate fully with the security department in enforcing the parking regulations.

Buildings

All buildings of the facility should be diagrammed and their security needs analyzed. This analysis should include, particularly, requirements for key control, alarms, protective lighting, stairwells and escape routes, location of emergency equipment, and security of shipping and receiving areas.

Specialized Interior Locations

A list of areas with special requirements should be made, with pertinent and practical recommendations regarding fire, theft, crowd control, and specified emergencies. Basically, specific areas of concentration to be included are:

Administrative offices
Animal storage
Cafeteria/Coffee shop
Canteen areas
Cashiers' offices
Closed circuit TV locations
Communications equipment
Data processing department
Dietary department
Document storage (prescription blanks, visitors' passes, etc.)
Emergency department
Employees' lockers, lounge area, and entrances
Flammable substance storage
Fire exits, equipment
Geriatrics department
Gift shop
Heating and air conditioning systems
Housekeeping department
Intensive care department
Laundry room
Lost and found
Lounge areas
Mail room
Maintenance department
Medical library
Nursing offices/Residences
Obstetrics department
Operating rooms
Outpatient clinics
Pathology lab, morgue, and specimen storage
Patient property
Patrol (routes and scheduling)
Pediatrics department
Personnel (identification)
Pharmacy (hospital drug store)
Physicians' examination room
Physicians' mail room
Psychiatric department
Record storage (patient, x-ray)
Recovery rooms

Research and development areas
Respiratory therapy departments
Security headquarters
Supply, nonpharmaceutical
Supply, pharmaceutical

Physical Changes

A complete breakdown of physical changes in your existing facility, changes that are required to implement each phase of the survey's recommendations, must be presented. Additionally, the projected cost for such changes must be itemized realistically. Where possible, two or three alternatives should be furnished.

Fire Prevention and General Safety

This section of the checklist should list comprehensive suggestions for fire prevention and fighting, including location of emergency exits, methods of evacuation, and methods of summoning the fire department. Included also should be recommendations concerning fire drills and classes to teach fire prevention to all employees. Similar recommendations should cover other emergency situations, including bomb threats, natural disasters, power failures, etc. Separate emergency manuals should be drawn up and distributed to department heads, who should be responsible for instructing their employees as to the proper methods for evacuation.

This section should also advise the administrator of an effective method for instructing personnel in general safety measures and ridding the facility of areas deemed unsafe due to improper storage of materials, traffic congestion, poor lighting and ventilation, etc.

Theft

Recommendations should be fully detailed concerning all vulnerable areas of inhouse and outside theft of materials, medicines, etc. Of course, as is the case in any large company, in any hospital theft will occur regardless of the amount of built-in controls. But it can be monitored and checked by an honest, competent security director who receives the administration's full and continual backing at all times and in all circumstances.

Personnel Requirements/Staff Composition

Here the survey should enumerate specific requirements regarding security personnel: training, experience, etc. If the staff is to be your own rather than that of an agency, you must have absolute control over the training program and the daily performance standards of the force. I have personally dealt with both staff security and agency security, and prefer staff security. Although, on the surface, each system appears to have attributes, the day-to-day frustrations of agency dealings must, of necessity, negate their use. You pay the agency a *contract* price for overall services; therefore, you cannot easily monitor and correct an individual staff member's continual failure to perform. You lose many aspects of pinpointed control. The agency does take many items off your hands: uniforms, taxes, insurance, bookkeeping, scheduling, hiring, firing, etc. But your per-hour payment for either staff or agency security is relatively the same, and in the case of staff security, you have full control. You are the direct employer, you dictate and monitor training and performance standards, and your own staff generally feels loyalty to you as the employer rather than to an intermediary agency. And your own staff can be provided with effective leadership and controls through a qualified inhouse security director, who in turn maintains continual contact with management.

Conclusion

I cannot overemphasize the importance of an all-inclusive security survey, conducted by a professional consultant who can readily spot and interpret problems and outline practical, but cost-effective solutions. In reviewing the consultant's findings, you must check and recheck the expenditures of your existing system and compare them to the proposed revised system. Do not merely compare dollars to dollars; carefully weigh the comparative expenditure/product ratios. For example, a minimum per-hour wage payment does not necessarily mean that you *cannot* get good staff members, but it very definitely will affect the intensity of their training and experience. Too many administrators look at the expended dollars without checking their return. Here, a consultant and your inhouse security director can save you money while it might appear they are spending it.

The complete professional survey should furnish you with all itemized requirements and related costs. Under no circumstances should you accept the advice of the security consultant regarding use of a specific agency; the consultant's knowledge is useful, but an independent investigation and decision remain mandatory.

Part II
Security Systems and Controls

Chapter 3

Physical Security: Monitoring Access to Buildings and Grounds

The most effective system in the world, the most astute policies, and the most workable procedures will not work without discipline. The hospital administrator must therefore support completely every security policy, procedure, system, and control; where necessary, such support must include termination of the offending employee.

Systems and controls must begin at the architectural stage, through the consultative authority of the security director. Many dollars will be saved if the director knows the security business and starts operating at this stage. Fences, gates, enclosures, lighting, access roads, traffic requirements, alarms, locks, surveillance equipment, etc., should be carefully planned. No item of any nature should be allowed to move into, through, or out of the facility without the full knowledge and control of the director of security, and within the framework of the systems and controls then in effect.

All policies and procedures must be in writing and issued to all concerned. The policies must not only point out what shall be done, but must also indicate what corrective action will be taken for any failure to comply. It is essential that prior to publication every new policy and procedure be routed to each and every department head for perusal and comments. A failure to follow this simple rule will lead not only to failures of the procedures, but also to misunderstanding and perhaps resentment. Routing of new policy can be accomplished by a "bucksheet" method, whereby each department head must reply by a cutoff date or be assumed in agreement with the new policy or procedures as written.

Although policies, procedures, systems, and controls should be published to cover every conceivable area of the operation, security systems must control, but never dominate or interfere with facility operation. Therefore, all new policies must be continually reappraised during an initial operating or "trial" period to assure that they in fact solve the problem for which they were designed. Here again, failure to follow this simple rule will lead to disaster and extra cost. In addition, all security personnel must be thoroughly briefed concerning new policy to prevent confusion and, more potentially dangerous, a poor reaction to an unexpected situation. If personnel understand all ramifications of policy, you are preparing the facility and staff for planned *action* in response to a problem rather than unauthorized *reaction.*

BUILDING CONTROLS

It must be kept in mind at all times that all controls must be *absolute.* Any relaxation of or deviation from any control automatically nulls that control. Building controls must be in effect for personnel, vehicles, equipment, supplies, keys, documents, etc. The sophistication of these controls must be dictated by security requirements as well as budget. But any control should be realistically budgeted so that it can be utilized fully. For example, in a key control system, the budgetary shortcut of inadequate records does not constitute control of those keys.

Personnel Identification

Both the standard and sophistication of the personnel identification system must be the highest possible. This control system must include all persons, regardless of stature. Color-coded ID cards have proven to be the most effective method of personnel control. Here again, the administrator must be wary of security consultants who promote a shortcut method that appears cheaper. In the long run, the better bargain will be the system that calls for a larger initial investment, but that effectively controls personnel entrance into the facility and access to high-risk areas. Your specific requirements are the best basis upon which to work; but you must not accept an unsophisticated system, such as one utilizing a numbered metal disk in place of a color-coded card, because you have "only five employees." Experience has shown, and I believe will continue to show, that the five employees could readily become fifty, then five hundred, and so on. It is therefore imperative that, regardless of how small the facility, you establish a system of personnel control as if you were in the process of controlling 500-plus people.

According to the requirements of the facility, card coding must be instituted at the outset. With the entire card one color, you can add, when requirements demand, other colors, stripes, and/or graphic designs that will facilitate instant recognition regarding employee department and limited or full facility access. Colors could stand for specific departments, buildings, floors, etc. As an example, if a floor has three different areas requiring three different access rules, access to all areas of the floor could be recognized by the use of an all-blue card; a blue card with one diagonal black stripe could identify access to Area 1 only, with two black stripes for access to Area 2 only, and three black stripes for access to Area 3 only. Naturally, any coding can be applied, but to facilitate operation, it must be simple and sensible.

The identification card would also provide photo identification for all permanently assigned personnel; a simple, but coded card should also be issued to all visitors, vendors, and other authorized nonpersonnel when they enter the building. Where necessary and advisable, it is a simple matter for the permanent employee's identification card to become a key to the employee parking area and interior locked passages, and even to actuate time records for pay purposes. The information to be recorded on the identification card should be brief, but effective. Extraneous information, such as home address, telephone number, etc., which has no bearing on the individual's identity at the time identity is questioned for building security, should be left off the card. Should such information ever be necessary during a security check, the security guard can call the 24-hour manned security office, where detailed records of all employees are filed.

The issuance and return of any means of employee identification must be completely controlled by the security department. Facility regulations must demand an exit interview, which is as essential as an entrance interview, and must include individual clearance from the security department. (Additional controls regarding personnel are discussed in Chapter 4.)

Staff Parking

Management must take a very "hard-nosed" attitude toward vehicle controls. Where repeated or flagrant violations of the vehicle control policy are found, management must be ready and willing to take severe disciplinary action to ensure the program's effectiveness. When the policies are not followed, havoc in the parking area will undoubtedly result. The program of employee parking requires very close cooperation from all members of the facility. Where necessary, complete explanations regarding the restrictions must be published and given to all. Where feasible, the personnel manager should attempt to encourage or form car pools to help alleviate parking problems.

Because the controlled parking area is, of course, most desirable, registration of vehicles should be mandatory. All new employees should immediately register their vehicles with security in order to receive assigned parking spaces. Although costly from the worker-hours point of view, parking assignment works; the assignment of choice parking spots is a great morale builder, and older employees work to enforce the parking program. Choice spots could be assigned on a points basis as well as the standard seniority basis, with points being awarded or lost on the basis of frequency of parking or other traffic violations. For easy and instant recognition of parking privileges, each employee should be provided with a windshield sticker or other identifying label.

One of the problems involved in parking programs in the inevitable damage to vehicles. The majority of parking lot accidents are minor, resulting in mere scratches. Most are the result of straight-in parking. Although angle parking does take up perhaps one extra parking space per row, headaches and damages will be held to a minimum. Angle parking also aids traffic flow.

The problem of whether to station a guard in the parking lot should have been covered and answered by your professional consultant's survey. If it does not seem cost-effective to have full-day, stationary coverage, perhaps a roving patrol will prove desirable to check for damage, flat tires, leaking gas tanks, lights left on, etc. Aided by the identifying windshield sticker, the security department can relay such information to the employee for immediate action.

Management should recognize that the employee morale and safety resulting from efficient vehicle control is a cost-effective reason to establish such control. Low or bad morale can cost dollars in reduced work performance. Employee benefits should include a restricted parking area protected by security. Employee cars and accessory equipment are fine theft targets. For safety reasons, the parking areas should be located as close to the employee entrance as possible. And in a medical facility, since many of the employees are women, special precautions should be taken to avoid violent personal crime. It is my belief, especially in view of today's employment market, that employees must be pampered. If they are not, they will go elsewhere.

Key Control

The key control system must be absolute, and it must be controlled by the security department. No key control system is complete unless the keys for the facility are given directly to the director of security before the initial locks are installed. The lock installation should be done by the director or the director's bona fide assistant, and under no circumstances should any of the keys be allowed out of the hands of security until installation of the locks is complete. In any key control system, loss of control occurs when keys are distributed. The secret to retaining control is extremely simple: Do not issue any keys! I realize the rashness of this statement and that it is certainly necessary to issue keys to certain people. But you must understand that as soon as keys are issued, the key control system and the security of the facility has been breached insofar as those particular keys are concerned.

Under no circumstances should more than one grand master key be issued; it should be in the hands of only the director of security. Although it might seem that the administrator, senior physicians, and surgeons should each have keys, there are several very good security reasons why they shouldn't. Since the security director would not presume to enter the operating room and proceed to interfere, so members of the facility should not attempt to interfere in the efforts of security. There has yet to be a facility that has not had a breach of its key control system by virtue of the fact that a master key and a grand master key were issued to personnel other than security. There is no sense in spending thousands of dollars on locks and keys only to have the system thwarted by one unthinking individual.

There are several types of key control systems. A master key system is by far the best. It should go into effect from day one and should remain in effect under the complete control of security. Should you have a master key system in effect at the time you hire a security director who feels that the system has been compromised or is otherwise less than adequate, it will be to your advantage to consider the reasoning and recore the entire facility, even though such a move will inevitably cost more money initially. But under no circumstances should any key control system or planning for a master key system be made by anyone other than a qualified security consultant.

You will be able to determine your new security director's worth by virtue of the demand made concerning recoring the entire facility. If your director does not make this demand, I suggest that you hire yourself another. No responsible person will accept the job of security director of any facility that has a master key system without personal and complete control of the keys. If not given the permission to recore, due to facility budgetary restrictions, the director will insist that the request for recoring be made a matter of record and that any occurrence resulting from the key control system in effect at the time will not be his or her responsibility.

Of primary importance in a master key system is the service received after the system has been installed. Every key company or lock company will promise the moon at the time you are about to sign a contract. However, after the contract has been signed and the system installed, the service aspect may be sadly neglected. A key and lock company must provide certain services. There are several well-known companies that offer interchangeable cores and master key systems: I recommend the Best Lock

Corporation of Indianapolis. Through their various area representatives, they offer what they term the "I package." I recommend it because:

1. A systems expert analyzes your present and future locking requirements.
2. Your locks are master keyed by faultless mathematics, within the original plan approved by you. The complete line of locks, for every purpose, are products of the very best materials and workmanship.
3. As further protection, Best delivers locks and keys only upon your written authorization and identification. Also, receipts show that the locks and keys were delivered directly to you. The codes to your combination are maintained under tight security at their plant.
4. Materials and workmanship of all Best products are fully guaranteed, and aid from the systems experts is always available directly from the factory.

One must realize the vast importance of the various keys that constitute a master key system. The *grand master key* will open any lock in the entire facility; the *master key* will open any lock in a particular series; the *submaster key* will open any lock in a subseries; the *operating* or *change key* will open an individual lock; and the *core key* will change the cores of the locks. It stands to reason that if you are in possession of the core key and any operating or change key, you need only remove and change the individual core that fits your key and the core of the lock on the door to which you desire access. This is accomplished by using the core key to remove the existing core and replacing it with a new one. But if you as administrator allow this changing process to be handled by the maintenance department instead of security, you are, in effect, handing maintenance a grand master key, since in the future no lock will be safe from anyone who has access to the core key. Therefore, to emphasize: In a key control system, security and security alone administers to any and every need with regard to the locking requirements of the facility. When a lock has to be installed or removed, or when a core has to be changed, the security department must do it.

Control must be present over each block-set core and key as well as the door or closure in which the lock set is installed. Such control must, of course, be absolute and must start at the time the system is installed. A haphazard manner of handling any part of the system will automatically void the system in its entirety, thus providing the facility with an extremely costly, insecure security investment. From the outset, then, you must carefully plan exactly where a key is really needed and how many duplicate keys are needed. Many employees and department heads will advise you that they each need a key; they might have a thousand good excuses. Obviously, unless there is a bona fide reason, no key should be issued. And a reasonable review of your actual requirements, not those you inherit from an old, inefficient system, will show you that the need to issue keys is, in fact, very small. Your review will quickly show that all places "needing" keys and locks in fact do not. The same applies to people needing keys.

The use of security officers at guard stations and entrances will further reduce need of locks and keys, and may save money, assuming that guards are not overused. Doors that require continual access during routine work hours need not be furnished with locks and keys requiring daily issue. Instead, your security officer could open and close these doors at specified times. By scheduling and assigning your security officers in conjunction with your key requirements, you can reduce key issuance needs to almost nil. But to have a guard stand eight hours in front of a door merely to open that door when needed is a waste of money. By use of closed-circuit television and electrically controlled doors, you can easily cover an entire facility and its routine locking needs with one guard. Such coverage gives you unequalled security at places requiring special precautions, such as drug centers and cash offices. Such areas, which require entry and exit at varying times by various people, can be controlled by the use of a double type of lock and a remote-control television. Any number of card keys could be issued to any number of individuals. Use of the card keys would automatically record who opened which door at what time. That is, it would record the name of the person to whom the card was issued; it would not necessarily identify the actual person using the card. But at the time that the door was to be opened, the insertion of the card key would alert a security officer some distance away, who would, by remote control television, determine whether or not the person had authorized access. By then pressing a button, the security guard would open the door. Should the person wanting to enter be unauthorized, the security guard could take whatever steps were necessary. Use of a master key by the individual seeking entry would, of course, bypass this system, but upon insertion of the key, the alarm would still alert the guard who would then verify the individual's access authority. Close scheduling would be required to avoid the possibility of collusion between guard and offender. Automatic records not under the control of either the security officer or the person using the assigned key would also have to be maintained. But the savings in wage dollars, the increase in efficiency of facility operation, the increase in security coverage, and the increase in the life of your key control system, will very soon add up to offset the cost involved in installing and using the combination of television cameras, alarms, guards, and locks.

Your administrative review of the key control system should, of course, start upon your acceptance of the security responsibility for the facility. Such review may show that areas of the facility, if moved, could not only furnish better facility security, but better overall efficiency. Review the existing blueprints; include every door, present and anticipated. Every door in the facility should be numbered, regardless of whether it needs a lock or not. Thus, if a free-swinging door is later changed to a locked door, it will not ruin your numbering system. An open archway should also be included in the numbering system as if it were equipped with a door. If the numbers are to be attached physically to the doors, the door frames containing the doors should also be numbered, in case the doors themselves are moved from one location to another. This will assure that the numbering sequence remains in chronological order throughout the facility; even if doors and locks are moved.

Key issuance should be handled only by the director of security or the director's assistant and must not be relegated to any other person. All keys and cores should be physically locked in a metal cabinet in the security director's office, which in turn should be locked. Access should be limited to the director.

The key control system depends upon records. Although at planning time it may not appear to be necessary, good security and insurance against the compromise of the system will demand that such records be maintained. All records must be kept under lock and key in the security director's office at all times, and maintained by the director. Records could be kept on color-coded index cards, showing: key number, door number, core changes, door change authorizations, key holder, core number, requests for keys and/or cores.

It is absolutely imperative that the director of security and the director's assistant be the only people possessing a grand master key and a core key. Under no circumstances should these keys ever be allowed out of their possession. Only they should be allowed to order keys and/or cores, and to sign for their receipt. Such authorization and receipt should be in effect from the start of construction or time of takeover by the new security director. In addition, no type of major maintenance should be undertaken without the full approval of the security director if such maintenance will have any effect whatsoever on key control.

Chapter 4

Internal Financial Security: Protection against Theft and Mismanagement

THE DISHONEST EMPLOYEE

Because of its unfortunate frequency, internal dishonesty is an all-too-familiar topic to management. Statistics in cases I have investigated show that internal staff were responsible for approximately 75 percent of all facility theft, and that management-level personnel were responsible for the greater part of that theft. And unlike fire losses, losses from employee theft which may equal or exceed fire losses, are generally not covered by insurance. In brief, the internal thief can very easily turn an otherwise profitable enterprise into a prime candidate for bankruptcy.

Weak Spots and Criminal Motivation

A survey of your facility will show the areas obviously vulnerable to theft, such as supply rooms, cash drawers, cafeterias, gift shops, etc. Common sense dictates strict security in these areas. (Other, less obvious areas will be discussed later in the chapter.) A good starting place in curbing facility theft is the conscientious application of *control* in all vulnerable areas. Just as leaving the ignition keys in a parked car might motivate a person to steal the car, so might a relaxed system of control over a supply area motivate otherwise trusted employees to help themselves.

The three necessary elements to a criminal act are motive, opportunity, and means. Although management can put various restraints on each, only *opportunity* can be controlled. Motives can be curbed by an effective program of positive morale building and company loyalty and built-in reminders of the consequences of illegal acts. The means to steal can be controlled to a certain extent by routine checks at various doors, and by limiting employee access to high-risk areas. But the internal thief, aware of facility policy regarding door checks, will still manage to circumvent the system by getting stolen items out through "secured" doors. Therefore, the only controllable element is opportunity. It will diminish significantly with effective controls.

It is impossible to list all the things that might trigger an employee theft. However, experience shows that the following individuals have the most opportunities:

1. Supervisors and other authority figures
2. Guards
3. Night and weekend employees who are generally unsupervised for long periods
4. People with keys
5. Long-time trusted employees
6. Storekeepers and receivers
7. Clerks handling money and payroll or equipment records
8. Service department personnel
9. Terminating employees

I include this list not to suggest guilt or to exclude other potential thieves, but to generalize the profile; keys, time, lack of supervision or accountability, and authorized access to materials and records represent opportunity. Twenty-five percent of all employees will steal to some degree if they feel they can get away with it, and only a very small percentage are ultimately caught. It is upsetting to note that within that 25 percent, the management-level thief is responsible for over 60 percent of the total loss.

Types of Internal Dishonesty

Embezzlement and Fraud

Embezzlers are successful primarily because they are respected employees who handle financial records. Embezzlement is the most costly white collar crime. One expert outlined that embezzlers leave their place of employment each working day with more than $8 million of employers' cash and merchandise, a total of more than $2 billion annually. Regular burglars and robbers do not do half as well. I happen to believe that the $2 billion figure is conservative. Many embezzlers are either not caught or, if caught, not prosecuted.

I know of a company that refused to pursue an embezzler because to do so might have caused a run on the finances of the company. The situation was not even reported to the insurance carrier for the same reason. Thus the stockholders paid the loss, which was in the thousands of dollars, by getting a decreased dividend. Naturally, they were not aware of the situation. And such a case represents the synergistic compounding of crime: the embezzlement, unexposed by management, led to the further crime of fraud to the stockholders.

An effective security system will reveal embezzlement before it becomes disastrous. The use of security audits and document control, discussed later in this chapter, has proven highly effective in my experience. But additionally, management can make itself aware of suspicious signs. Always be suspicious of those who vehemently oppose change, particularly if such change would place restrictions on them or on their known friends or relatives. Always monitor the "model" employees who are never late and who do not take days off or vacations. If you have employees who are charged with taking care of all aspects of a transaction and who declare that their jobs are more important than any vacation, watch them closely. In reality, the chances are good that they are worried about being caught if others are assigned, even temporarily, to do their jobs.

Remember that embezzlers steal billions because they know how to make the documents appear correct. When was the last time you really checked the records of transactions you have allowed others to handle? By "really check," I mean all copies of the involved documents, not merely the copy sent to your office.

Management must also be aware of the danger involved in hiring relatives or close friends of other key employees. A recent case of fraud, uncovered by an efficient security system at a department store, involved a payroll clerk and her husband, who was hired as temporary seasonal help in the stockroom. When the season was over, he was terminated. However, the security system soon revealed that, although he had factually ceased employment, he was still collecting a weekly pay check. Our subsequent investigation revealed that his wife had created false time cards for him, keeping him on the payroll records. When the payroll checks arrived at the store, she received all of them for disbursement, and merely removed the one for her husband before forwarding the remainder of the stockroom checks to the department head. Incidentally, the security system that caught her had been in effect for only one month; had the theft occurred over previous months, it would not have been exposed.

The foregoing is an example of relatively minor fraud and embezzlement; financial executives juggling figures and skimming funds are capable of creating far more dramatic losses to the company. But through effective security audits and document control, outlined later in this chapter, your security director can discourage and ultimately diminish such theft.

Sidetracking and Pilferage

Too many administrators fail to see the folly of stationing a guard at the front door of the facility to monitor members of the public who enter and leave, while leaving the employees' entrance and the shipping and receiving areas open with no security present at all. The amount of money that is lost through your front doors over a ten-year span will in no way match the loss you suffer in one year through your back doors. In general, the following represent materials most often vulnerable to employee pilferage:

1. Linens: sheets, towels, blankets, curtains, draperies
2. Clothing: uniforms, aprons, robes, and gowns
3. Food: patient trays, cafeteria and dietary department supplies
4. Maintenance supplies: paint, hardware, light bulbs, lumber, hand and power tools, plumbing supplies
5. Paper goods: stationary, office supplies, housekeeping supplies
6. Capital equipment: electric fans, projectors, typewriters, furniture, floor polishers
7. Drugs and pharmaceuticals
8. Money: facility and personal
9. Patients' and employees' belongings: jewelry, luggage, clothing, personal appliances
10. Medical supplies and equipment: stethoscopes, surgical instruments, laboratory equipment
11. Gift shop supplies and equipment
12. Housekeeping supplies: soaps, brooms, pails
13. Photographic supplies and equipment: cameras, film, projectors, enlargers
14. Time: intangible, but costly

The term "pilferage" usually means small-scale theft of insignificant items. However, regular or long-term pilferage will rapidly add up to a major loss. I therefore emphasize the need for security at all employee entrances, regular inventory of all materials, periodic checks on the procedures used to order and disburse materials, an effective system of package control, and, as in all areas of security coverage, complete cooperation from management in the investigation and apprehension of suspected thieves.

Sidetracking, although less frequent than pilferage, usually involves materials of greater value. The director of security, by periodically referring to company audits and reports can ensure a low percentage of sidetracking theft. While employed by a four-store retail chain, I devised a system that was used in one of the stores on a trial basis. These stores dealt in quality merchandise, netting between $35 million and $40 million per store per year. One of the more lucrative departments was, of course, television and stereo. The store management assigned a new manager to the television department. The new manager, a former salesman, had been watched by security for an ongoing period because he was suspected of theft. Unfortunately, in making the promotion, the store management did not consult with the security department. Nevertheless, within one month of his assignment, my system showed that he had made two illegal transactions whereby he was shipping televisions out of the store to a "fence," who in turn was selling them at a greatly reduced price. When we finished our investigation, we had uncovered that this man had, in one month and through only two transactions, removed some $12,000 worth of televisions and had even had the nerve to put in for his sales commission on the "sale" of the sets!

The system that caught this man was in operation in only one store; if we project the loss over four stores, you can readily see how badly this one company could be hit by dishonest employees. Incidentally, a year before, a member of the same department was apprehended and found to have been stealing very heavily over the preceding six years. His total theft was reported to be close to $500,000. One year later in another store, a theft in the television department was discovered, involving over $60,000, also going on for years. This same company sustained a loss of many thousands of dollars through a highly placed executive. Such organized thefts of major amounts of merchandise *can* be uncovered and diminished; again, a program of document control, equipment control, and security audit will more than pay for itself.

Kickbacks and Collusion

It must be understood that curbing facility theft includes not only preventing the taking of goods, but also monitoring attitudes and behavior patterns that, experience reveals, eventually *lead* to stealing. Here, information on the relationships among employees and between employees and outside suppliers is vital, since such information could foretell possible dishonesty by an otherwise trusted employee. Collusion can breed coercion can breed overwhelming losses.

Collusion, the cooperative meeting of two thieves, can be present anywhere in the facility. For example, it could involve a document falsification scheme between members of the shipping and accounting departments; it could involve an authorized keyholder's "loaning" keys to someone else; and it could involve a major kickback operation between the facility purchasing agent and an outside supplier.

The purchasing department requires special attention, as it is an area particularly vulnerable to kickback. In brief, management must monitor long-term relationships between inhouse purchasing agents and outside suppliers. Be wary of the agent who prefers to deal with an established supplier in any new transactions rather than to receive competitive bids; while in reality merely extending the kickback, the agent may argue that the established supplier's quality of service and fair prices are known. The unchallenged, long-term relationship can lead to many abuses. The supplier, now assured of business, becomes lax in the accounts. Orders may be neglected and quality reduced, while top-line materials are channeled to another facility where the purchasing agent is not on the take. It might be more profitable for the supplier to court the other company.

Another abuse of the purchasing department is the practice of accepting Christmas gifts and the like from outside suppliers. By allowing such gratuities to be accepted, management places the purchasing agent and/or other employees in a position of compromise. Because it has become accepted as a common practice, it is difficult to control. But discretion must be employed to ensure that such gifts do not create special interests; supply companies that do not offer gifts and favors must, of course, not be alienated. My point is obvious—management must stay actively involved and be willing to challenge when competition between suppliers appears suspiciously absent.

INTERNAL CONTROL SYSTEMS

No system has yet been created that can stop dishonest employees; we can temporarily slow them down, but as soon as they have figured out the new system of controls, they will find a way around it and be back in full swing again. It is therefore the job of the security staff to keep placing blocks in the paths of dishonest employees so as to spot them before they can do much damage.

Perhaps the greatest enemy of internal control is management. For whatever reason, facility management often tends to discourage or even prohibit the use of internal controls because of misplaced loyalty to employees whose own loyalty is debatable. At other times, management discourages internal controls because the cost seems exhorbitant. Sometimes objections are raised by respected executives who simply do not understand either the seriousness of the problem or the simplicity of the proposed control. In far too many instances, management vetos a program of internal control because a highly placed "trusted" employee suggests that the problems can be handled less expensively or more subtly;

sometimes it later develops that this employee is actually stealing from the company!

In such cases, an established, professional control system could eventually lead to uncovering the thief. As an example, I once had experience with the personnel director of a large company who had the responsibility of administering the employees' profit-sharing plan. Over the years, in his position of trust, he methodically diminished the funds of the plan and diverted them to his own use. This man continually fought all proposed new security policies, especially when they concerned new auditing procedures to be followed through by the security department. He knew that as each new procedure went into effect, the net would be closing in on his activities; sooner or later the security proposals would involve the checking of the profit-sharing plan that he was administering and from which he was stealing. His objections were vehemently put forth in written memos through official channels and verbally and unofficially over lunch with whomever would listen, particularly with people who had influence over security policies and procedures.

Management must realize the full implications of, and various motivations behind, advice that discourages the establishment of internal controls; effective security is not a luxury item, but a mandatory, cost-effective protection. Internal controls must combine published and enforced regulations with physical security devices; they must extend in coverage to include all equipment, furniture, fixtures, supplies, documents, etc. Associative controls covering the physical security of the facility buildings and grounds were covered in Chapter 3; the following sections concentrate on *internal* security involving personnel screening and potential financial loss involving money, equipment, and documents.

Personnel Screening and Follow-Up Investigations

Control over internal dishonesty must begin with comprehensive background investigations on all personnel hired. Since such an undertaking is relatively expensive, we must draw lines as to who should and should not be screened. Certainly all people hired for, or promoted to, a key position in which they shall directly handle expensive equipment (regardless of size), supplies, food, office equipment, money, drugs, etc. *must* be the subject of a background investigation. Security screening is especially important in mass hirings; when many people are needed quickly, selectivity and security checks are sometimes unfortunately allowed to lapse in the interest of expediency. This oversight can obviously cause problems.

Background investigations should be handled by staff investigators whenever possible, and by outside agencies only when staff investigators are not employed. (For a further discussion of the responsibilities of the internal investigatory staff, see Chapter 7.)

To ensure a comprehensive background investigation on incoming personnel, you must begin with a thorough employment application form. It must ask for a complete outline of former employment, including names of immediate supervisors. Experience has proven that the applicant who fails to complete an application is an applicant of whom you should be wary. The personnel department must be willing to rely on the security department to authenticate application form information; a qualified security investigator can more easily spot misinformation and/or misleading information than the average personnel interviewer.

An employer should, of course, never rely on resume information unless it is fully substantiated. There is probably false or misleading information on many of the resumes in your file. Failure to record information can constitute submission of false information. In my own security business, where every potential employee knows that we will check and double check, we still find that a very large percentage of the applications and resumes contain false information. The problem is that such documents are usually not fully checked until the questionable actions of the employee cause the employer to go *back* and check. Basically, falsification on a resume usually consists of the applicant's falsifying educational background or former job titles, and magnifying prior performance. Beware of vague descriptions of education, job title, and performance. Check every item on each form.

The usual background investigation conducted by most personnel departments is done by telephone or mail, and is too often extremely shallow, requiring only check marks as answers rather than detailed profile sheets. Also, due to the severity of civil laws, it is almost impossible to obtain adverse information on an individual. However, a qualified security director can at least ask the right, probing questions, and with facility security the principal motivation rather than the applicant's job-related quality, the security director can pinpoint behavioral trends that may have been considered less important to the personnel interviewer intent on concentrating on the applicant's *professional* attributes.

The security department should also conduct yearly follow-up investigations to monitor changes in the attitudes and action of employees. This is particularly necessary as reference file data if employees are being considered for a promotion. When promotions are considered, the security department should be notified in advance to submit updated files on the employee; those under consideration should not be advised of potential promotions until the updates are completed.

Information obtained from the updated security file would include a compendium of updated background data and current data on individuals' recent performance in their current positions. Such information could be adverse to individuals, but ultimately advantageous to the company. Security would naturally have to be trained and constantly reminded to gather only substantiated, accurate, and *relevant* information.

Each employee's updated security file must represent a cooperative effort between the security and personnel departments. If security comes across any proven information that is adverse to an individual, the director of security should immediately and personally inform the personnel manager in writing; the notification form should be in duplicate so that one copy remains in the personnel file and one copy returned to the security file, with the personnel manager's signature as indication of receipt. Under no circumstances should security or personnel release such information to other members of the staff unless the security department deems that related activity of the employee warrants action; in this case, management must be informed.

Cooperation between the personnel and security departments must be two-way; copies of all employee applications and any other documents affecting the status of each employee should be forwarded to security for their files, and personnel must consult with the security department on a frequent basis. The personnel department should fully understand how such an arrangement is beneficial to overall personnel management. As an example, if an employee suddenly decides to apply for insurance, confidential security information that would affect such coverage could prevent a potential insurance fraud. In addition if another company calls for a reference on an individual, the files held by the security department may provide adverse information concerning the employee.

Finally, each employee should be interviewed and cleared by security upon termination notification. It is unfortunately not uncommon that a disgruntled employee, or merely a terminating employee whose loyalties are in transition, plans a coup just before leaving; when the theft is discovered, that person is long gone and least suspected. Also, a fellow employee could become a source of stolen goods for a terminated employee. Another function of the security department interview with terminating employees is the return of all keys, identification cards, and so on.

Equipment Control

One of the greatest fallacies of business is that all kinds of controls, checks, and cross-checks are placed on cash, from petty cash on up, and yet very few controls are placed on equipment. Educating employees and management alike that a box of paper clips represents 50 cents and a computer terminal represents thousands of dollars is an integral part of internal control.

If you dropped 50 cents on the floor, you would immediately get down and search for it; a box of paper clips dropped behind a desk would gather dust. If you gave a clerk $500 in cash to go to the store to buy something, you would carefully select the person, then remind that person of the value of the cash being carried. You would worry about your cash until the clerk returned. Yet you will allow fairly free access to your purchase order book. The point is that internal controls treat all equipment and documents as cash.

Internal equipment controls must start at your purchase office and run, as nearly as possible, to the point when the item is actually issued for use. As an example, security should monitor the purchase, subsequent receipt, issuance, and use location of each typewriter; control should continue until final disposition of the machine. Records reflecting a complete history of each item would collectively constitute a running inventory of all facility equipment.

Management must be aware, through the security department checks, that no unnecessary or frill item is ordered and paid for by the facility and then removed permanently from the facility by the manager who ordered it. Every item purchased must be definitely needed.

Naturally, some equipment must be allowed to leave the facility temporarily. But effective programs of control must be instituted through an extension of the inventory and accounting of location and use. A simple system is to list each item on its own individual card, with such cards being filed at the main security desk. Authorized removal of any item would be formally approved by a responsible person, and the actual removal would have to be accomplished through the main security desk. At the time of removal, the authorization would be filed at the security desk, and the card covering the item would be pulled and refiled in a diary box for continuous surveillance until the return of the item. Upon return, the card would be replaced in its original file position. The removal authorization itself would be held in still another file and, upon return of the item, would be marked and returned to the authorization agent for disposition.

Security measures must also be instituted to control the contents of packages carried in and out of the facility by employees. Although it sounds extremely harsh, in areas of high risk, this must include any extraneous container not an acceptable and necessary part of the employee's work clothing and uniform. Handbags, lunch containers, and thermos bottles should not be allowed beyond the employee entrance. Instead, employees should be furnished lockers. In particularly vulnerable theft areas, there should be absolutely no reason for any employee to bring any type of package into the facility. If a credible reason arises, special passes, closely controlled at all times by security, must be issued and close scrutiny enforced. I am familiar with one case in which an employee removed thousands of dollars worth of merchandise, including a pair of binoculars and a microscope, by hiding them in his thermos bottle. He had simply removed the thermos tube from the shell of the bottle and wedged a shot glass into the bottle neck to hide the contents. I realize that this sounds rather far-fetched, but experience in security has proven to me that a person intent on stealing will devise incredibly ingenious schemes.

Potentially helpful in discouraging equipment pilferage is the posting of signs that advise that closed circuit televisions are in operation for the safety and protection of all who use the facility. Facility equipment particularly vulnerable to pilferage is listed on page 28. Material related to controls of narcotics and dangerous drugs appears in Appendices B and C.

Document Control

Document control is an area that is usually left untouched by so-called experts in security due to a very definite lack of knowledge about not only the importance of documents, but also the systems that can be applied to control them. As with all controls, document controls must be absolute and strictly and continually enforced. Before you can really understand the extreme need for document control, you must fully understand and appreciate what, in fact, constitutes a document.

For our purposes, a document is a form that has been completed and, by such completion, has created a change in the status of some person or thing. When you are dealing with the movement of merchandise such as furniture, fixtures, supplies, etc., the document moving such items becomes, in fact, worth the dollar amount of the cost of replacing the items being moved. It is the record of possession and location; without it, the merchandise is lost. If a document is falsified, material can be stolen. And more devastating than the monetary and material loss of merchandise is the threat to human life that falsification of drug issuance documents represents. When you have a machine or a supply of drugs worth thousands of dollars transferred to or within your facility, and any part of such shipment can be sidetracked, you can bet your life that sidetracking will take place, especially if large illegal profits can be made. And your records might show that the merchandise was successfully transferred without incident. Obviously, the records are inaccurate; but falsification is fairly easy to accomplish and very difficult to trace.

No business or facility that wants to stay out of the red can long afford not to control its documents with the same tenacity that it controls its cash.

A business's documents generally represent on a daily basis hundreds, if not thousands, of times the value of the actual dollars in cash on hand. Cash is strictly accounted for, to the penny, and is kept under lock and key, protected by sophisticated alarm systems, but documents are generally handled rather carelessly.

Too many administrators are lulled into a false sense of security by the knowledge that their important documents are multicopy number-controlled forms, and therefore cannot be changed without very easily being noticed. But let me remind you of a few basic facts. First of all, you order these forms from a printer. What is to stop someone else from doing the very same thing? It has been done on many occasions. Many forms are also quite easily duplicated on home presses. And with your multicopy set of documents, doesn't each individual copy go to an individual employee, department, or section? The key word is *individual*. Of the usual four copies involved, one stays in the book, one goes with the merchandise, one goes to the accounting department, and one is kept by the shipper; any one copy can be altered. Perhaps, if you have a slightly more sophisiticated system, you will have the receiving copy authenticated at the point of receipt and then forwarded to accounting. In any case, you do not have a system in which any one of the original copies is checked against *a very definite original*. Also, the chances are excellent that you allow crossouts, strikeovers, and other changes to be made on any copy of the document. Each of these bastardizations costs you money and acts to nullify the document upon which it appears. Also, the chances are that your overall system of handling your documents would enable a "known and trusted" employee to advise accounting that a certain copy of the document would no longer be sent to them because it was being rerouted through a particular manager's office at that manager's request. And they probably would believe it! After all, this is a trusted employee.

Some years ago, while associated with one of the largest department store chains in the country, I was instrumental in creating a document control system that ended up saving the company hundreds of thousands of dollars in the first year of the system's existence. Prior to installing this system, they operated with multicopied, proof-printed, numbered documents. As with all such systems, the numerical control soon faded into oblivion. This was soon accepted by all members of management, up to and including the auditors and board or directors, as a "business hazard" that had to be tolerated. But after many years of such operation *and* an incalculable loss, the company decided to change the method of shipping from use of an outside carrier to use of their own carrier. Since this appeared to be an opportune time, they finally relented and authorized the use of my document control system.

In my system, every document used to move the merchandise had to be obtained from security, and in turn had to be accounted for under the signature of the recipient. This person, in turn, had accountability for any further issuance of the document. Such control extended to the loading and trip sheets used by the driver. As each piece of merchandise was loaded onto the truck at the central warehouse, it was recorded on a shipping manifest and counted by security. When the manifest was complete, all copies of it were forwarded to the security officer on the dock. Here it was authenticated and a copy was then pulled and held by security. Another authenticated copy was forwarded by mail to the receiving store and still another copy was forwarded to the store along with the driver. The truck was sealed after receiving merchandise for five stores and was sent on its way with the loading and trip sheet. Instructions to all store security and the drivers included the order that *only* the store security officer could remove and replace the seal. The store security officer would count each piece against the shipping manifest and refuse any load if the seal was broken. If the count was wrong or the paperwork, which had been verified as clean at the warehouse, showed any erasures, crossovers, strikeouts, or changes of any kind, the store security would immediately call the home office.

Any violation was subject to load refusal and an on-the-spot call to my office to advise of such violation. The document copies that went to the store were authenticated by the store security officer and returned to my office via the driver, who had to turn in each sheet with the trip sheet. Individual entries on the loading and trip sheet itself served as further authentication. Upon return to my office, all documents were matched and checked against the copies of the documents that were pulled at the time of shipping. When found to be in order, the return store copy was stamped as approved and forwarded to the accounts payable department. The approved data were then fed into a computer, which had previously been fed the data as recorded on the shipper's copy. Quarterly, the computer would give a readout verification to be checked against the warehouse receiving report and the buyer's purchase-order reports. The system not only ensured honesty and efficient merchandise accounting, but also served as a foundation for a meaningful inventory.

Despite all the security built into this system, there were changes to copies of the forms. In one case, we found a total of fifteen crossovers and strikeouts on the original copy; some $75,000 worth of merchandise would have been lost had it not been for the system. And this is just one of over sixty similar documents used in the course of the day. In another instance involving a single chain, I discovered yearly losses of over $18 million caused by a lack of control over documents. In every case in which a document control system was put into effect, a savings equal to and even greater than the cost of the entire security department was realized.

For those unable to employ a full security force for document control, I recommend that at no time should you allow any one person to handle all of the receiving and shipping chores designed to produce factual accountability of merchandise. Have a second person, without prior knowledge of the count, perform the incoming or outgoing count and forward the figures to a third person. This third person should then record it and forward it to the accounting department for further recording and checking against pertinent records. Above all, question each and every strikeout, crossover, and erasure. Should any employee repeatedly make "mistakes" on documents involving materials flow, take appropriate disciplinary measures. In addition, ensure that your accounting department maintains a complete record on all prenumbered forms in use. When possible, periodically allocate a full day to checking all documents used within a given period of time; they represent the history of your materials accountability and *must* be precise.

Special precautions regarding document security in the event of fire or bomb detonation are discussed in Chapter 5, pages 53-58.

Petty Cash Control

Petty cash is often an area of abuse. Several facility departments often need petty cash funds, and control often lapses because the amount of capital involved seems, according to its terminology, "petty." But a knowledgeable thief can work a $50 petty cash fund into a sizeable side income.

Usually, the accounting department and auditors are interested only in balancing petty cash receipts with fund allotments and cash on hand. Control should also extend to the verification of the actual use of the money, regardless of how "petty" the expenditures seem. The use of IOUs or the casual borrowing from the funds should not be tolerated. Common petty cash fraud that responsible administration can control includes: unauthorized use for personal purchases, alteration of receipts to falsify actual amount spent, and fabrication of receipts for articles never purchased or already purchased with other funds.

Payroll Control

Payroll control, from time card to paycheck, is often overlooked. All employees must account individually and personally for each actual hour that they work. Time clocks and time cards must always be positioned so that they can be closely supervised. Payroll control must be strictly enforced. It must be established facility policy that the "punching" of any time card other than one's own is grounds for immediate dismissal. (An alternative to the standard time card, the employee identification card, which is an extremely effective security device, is discussed in Chapter 3.)

Payroll records must be the subject of complete and continuing audit; a computer may facilitate the operation, but all figures should be cross-checked manually to avoid a costly long-term computer error. "Ghost payrolling" is one of the most lucrative ways that personnel and payroll clerks use to steal thousands of dollars. A good ghost payroller can continue for several years without being caught. Your only protection is an effective continuing audit of all payroll and personnel records.

The Security Audit

Even a small security department can effect some degree of control over materials mismangement and/or pilferage by monitoring the company records of material flow and by working in cooperation with the company auditors. I do not believe that the facility auditors should be given the sole responsibility of determining the amount of, and the facts surrounding, a loss due to materials mismanagement. In thirty years of experience I have yet to find an auditor with enough security knowledge to handle a complete investigation efficiently. Therefore, it is imperative that auditors and security staff combine efforts, and security must be allowed free access to all company records. In addition, the security department must answer directly to top management. In far too many companies, the security department is under the complete control of the personnel director, a system that can foil the objectivity and effectiveness of the auditing process. The personnel department, as well as all other departments, must be included in the security audit.

In order for any security audit system of property control to be effective, it must be all-encompassing. The security director must be made aware of every new capital purchase and every ultimate disposition of property. The security audit, if complete, will form an ideal facility inventory; all matters pertaining to each piece of property, its history and use location, will be available in one central place at all times.

Obviously, there are many other reasons why a security audit of all facility property is worth its cost. Identification and itemization of each item can aid in future insurance claims, accurate tax accounting, discouragement of employee theft, proper maintenance scheduling of machines and appliances, long-range planning of replacement schedule estimates, etc.

The actual responsibility for the program can rest with the accounting department, with the security department maintaining control. Audit review and update should be conducted on a regular basis throughout each facility department; but by "regular" I do not mean *scheduled*. In order to be truly effective, it should be unannounced.

Each piece of property should be properly identified by a numbered metal name plate affixed to it. The number would then be cross-referenced to a master number list as well as an alphabetized and departmentalized property list. I have found the "autograph" metal name plates to be among the best. These may be obtained from Metal Craft, Inc., Mason City, Iowa, or their local distributor in your area. In New England they are represented by the Bay State Calendar Co., Wellesley Hills, Massachusetts.

Proper organization of the actual audit process will require the cooperation of several people. A detailed procedure should be established, published, and enforced as company policy. Key individuals should be informed in a memo in which you:

1. outline the objectives and importance of property control
2. describe the use of the record forms
3. establish a uniform system of installation of permanent identification tags
   Suggestions:
   a. machinery: prominent, eye-level, on front if possible
   b. desks, tables, etc.: left side of back, immediately below top
   c. files, bookcases: front upper left-hand corner
   d. chairs: rear edge of seat or center of back
   e. warehouse trucks, etc.: prominent position, yet not where subject to being removed or defaced by movement or wear
4. assign responsibility for installing and maintaining the system

When establishing the audit inventory procedure, consider the future of the program as well as the present requirements. Decide what is required now and what might be required by property records as the facility expands. The following is an outline of various functions to be covered:

I. Physical Control
   A. Identification/ownership
   B. Location
   C. Custody
   D. Maintenance and repair records
II. Tax Accounting
   A. Original cost date—reconcile with actual conditions
   B. Depreciation method

    C. Group accounts or units
       1. Straight line
       2. Sum of life
       3. Declining balance
       4. Guidline lives
       5. Determined reserve ratios
III. Corporate Accounting
    A. Verification of asset values
    B. Cost accounting
    C. Distribution of overhead burden
IV. Fire Insurance
    A. Replacement cost (new/adjusted)
    B. Evidence of value
    C. Items excluded from coverage
 V. Plan for capital expenditures (near and long-term)
    A. Tax considerations
       1. Investment tax credit
       2. Guideline lives
    B. General considerations (moves, etc.)
    C. Equipment leased and/or purchased (list of all pertinent facts for each item)
       1. Inventory number
       2. Description
       3. Location
       4. Date of purchase/lease
       5. Cost (acquisition and installation)
       6. Depreciation (cost, method, and provision)
       7. Unrecovered cost
       8. Estimated remaining life
       9. Investment credit
      10. Asset classification

The actual decision as to what should be included in the property audit must rest with you. I highly recommend that every piece of property be inventoried by the system. For each item an individual card should be created, classified by asset category, listing:

Equipment number	Uncovered costs
Description	Estimated remaining life
Location	Investment credit
Date of purchase/lease	Depreciation method
Cost of acquisition/installation	Depreciation provision
Depreciation reserve	

All records and the item numbering system should be kept short and unencumbered. Numbering should be sequential and, unless absolutely necessary, uncoded. Only simple codes to identify specific locations, billing dates, etc., should be added to the numbering system, and should be simply indicated by use of a letter preceding the number. Such coding could also be indicated by different color identification plates.

Undercover Agents and Informers

Undercover agents can be hired through an outside agency and placed on your payroll as regular employees to oversee the activities of their "colleagues" and make daily reports to their supervisors. The use of such agents in vulnerable areas of theft might appear, superficially, to be highly beneficial. However, in actual practice it is often not cost-effective; agents are extremely expensive. I have personally used undercover agents in companies for which I was responsible for security, and after expenditure of many thousands of dollars, I found that the efforts of the agents netted me a return of 88 cents!

As in any outside agency dealings, the hospital administrator must be wary of the claims of a detective agency attempting to place undercover agents in the facility. The agency will have "facts" and figures that should be taken with a very large grain of salt; obviously, references should be demanded and checked thoroughly. An experienced security director or outside professional consultant can aid in the necessary weeding process. If the undercover agents of a particular agency are ultimately hired, the administrator must demand in the contract that the hospital's inhouse security director have absolute control over the agents and receive the agents' unedited daily reports directly. A copy of these reports should also go to the administrator.

Another means of employee surveillance is the use of the informer, your own employee who keeps you advised through daily reports to the security director. Informers are motivated by any number of reasons; unfortunately, money or revenge, rather than loyalty, are sometimes the motivating factors. Naturally, when selecting an informer, your best choice would be the individual motivated by loyalty. And even if the informer seems objective, any leads that he or she furnishes must be investigated by the security director before any subsequent action is taken. The truly professional security director will immediately spot the "stroker" and take whatever corrective action seems necessary.

The effectiveness of a voluntary informer system depends to a large extent on the rapport that the security staff has with the employees. However, much to our disadvantage, we find that the job performance of the majority of security personnel, even at the supervisory level, does not elicit the necessary respect that is the larger part of rapport. To compensate for a lack of voluntary informers, several facilities have turned to a reward program. The informer's reward must be large enough, and must also be given without any type of argument about whether or not the reward was actually earned. Obviously, you shouldn't just give the money away. However, don't quibble about technicalities. If ambiguities in the reward regulations create questions or problems, the mistake is that of management, and the employee must be paid. Nothing will kill a program faster than the complaints of an employee who performed but failed to get paid.

The identity of all informers must remain strictly confidential; you must be able to assure them that they will remain "silent witnesses" to any activities they may report. Careless treatment of their confidentiality could result in great harm to them.

Use of the informer rather than the undercover agent has several obvious benefits; the informer is your own employee, usually someone already accepted by the other employees. The undercover agent, on the other hand, must apply for the job and begin to build peer acceptability, a relatively lengthy process during which you are paying for surveillance and actually receiving little or nothing. Further, if the agent is spotted, and is therefore able to relay no information or is being used as conduit of false information, your investment will be not only costly but worthless. Certainly an inhouse informer could also be exposed, but if your security director is capable and professional, such exposure will occur far less frequently than agent exposure, and will not involve the large investment of time and money.

Bonding

Bonding represents an overall preventive measure against dishonest employees. In my experience, bonded personnel are far less apt to commit thefts and misappropriation. Any employee who handles stock or has authority or responsibility over items that represent real monetary value should be bonded.

In the event of a loss in which bonded personnel are involved, the insurance carrier will demand that you cooperate in the establishing of the settlement, as outlined in the bonding contract. The main problem involved will be "proof of loss." An efficient security department with established programs of equipment, monetary and document control will automatically fulfill this obligation for you. Without such controls, your claimed loss can compound itself in the form of wasted time and the possible subsequent cancellation by your insurance carrier.

I have had experience on both sides, as insurer and insured. As an insurance adjuster, I became well aware of the technicalities used to allow the insurance company to refuse to pay on a loss. And as an investigator for a company suffering the loss of a trailer truck loaded with merchandise, I have seen the other side. My investigation in this particular case revealed that our entire system of merchandise accountability did little more than generate paper. The theft and our subsequent realization of the sytem's inadequacies did, in the long run, help the company. However, our failure to "prove the loss" resulted in a loss in excess of $150,000; we could not be sure of the exact figure since the inadequate materials accountability documents could not even show us exactly what had been on the truck at the time it was stolen!

If a firm is paying the high price of bonding many employees, there is the danger of paying more to the bonding company over a period of years than it could possibly lose to theft during the same period. A good insurance company can figure the exposure, the number of people involved, and the amounts to be considered. The Surety Association of America in New York City, for example, will gladly supply, at no charge, formulation studies that can be used to determine the amount of bonding needed, based on the scope of your own particular facility.

Blanket Bonds

If there are a large number of employees to be bonded, a blanket fidelity bond, of which there are two kinds, is recommended. The *commercial blanket bond* covers all officers and employees collectively and, in the event of a loss, regardless of the number of employees involved, the aggregate amount collectible is the bond penalty. The bond is issued in a minimum penalty of $10,000; there is no maximum. The *blanket position bond* also covers all employees, but in the event of a collusive theft, the bond penalty applies to each employee involved in the loss. This bond has a minimum penalty of $2,500 and a maximum of $100,000. Both forms of bonds automatically cover all new employees during the term of the bond, without notice to the surety and without additional premium charge.

Schedule Bonds

If there are several bondable employees, a schedule form of bond would be advisable. There are two types of schedule bonds. The *name schedule bond* covers the individual employees by the name in amounts individually specified. This is similar to an individual bond; but, as a group policy, it covers more than one individually named employee. The *position schedule bond* provides protection against dishonest employees by position rather than by name, with coverage stipulated by individual position. In other words, the incumbent to a designated position within the company— book-keeper, treasurer, etc.— is automatically bonded. Thus, if three successive individuals occupy the position of bookkeeper during the life of the name schedule bond, a new acceptance specifying the amount of liability assumed must be obtained for each incumbent. Under the position schedule bond, however, the position of bookkeeper is bonded; therefore, no change is needed, regardless of the number of individuals who may hold that position during the term of the bond.

Conclusion

The actual type and amount of internal controls that should be instituted against dishonesty and mismanagement are, of course, matters for study at the particular facility. Basically, controls must be in force in all vulnerable areas to make pilferage and large theft impossible or, at least, extremely difficult. Further, the presence of controls should be publicized so that all potentially dishonest employees are made aware that they are running a risk.

All controls should be checked to ensure that, once installed, they are effective. If you as administrator can, in a test case, foil a control, is it because you are aware of an unpublicized pivot point of control, or is the control itself ineffectual?

All vulnerable areas in the facility must be thoroughly analyzed prior to control installation. Estimates of potential loss due to theft must be weighed against the proposed control costs. Obviously, six guards, an electric gate, and a man-eating Doberman to protect your paper clips would not be a wise investment.

Chapter 5

Emergency Security: Prevention and Control of Disasters

The program of emergency security encompasses both general safety measures, mandated by the William Steiger Occupation and Safety Health Act of 1970 (OSHA), and a comprehensive emergency preparedness program.

GENERAL SAFETY MEASURES

OSHA Requirements

The OSHA regulations, Public Law 91-596 of the 91st Congress, S219J, dated December 29, 1970, states in Section 5, which outlines duties, that "each employer shall furnish to each of his employees, employment, and place of employment which are free from recognized hazards that are causing or are likely to cause death, or serious physical injury, and comply with occupational, safety and health standards promulgated under this act." It is clear that the onus is upon the employer to rid the place of employment from hazards that may adversely affect the general safety and well-being of the employees. Further, the OSHA "Record Keeping Requirements" mandate that as of July 1, 1971, every employer who is covered under this act must keep occupational, injury, and illness records for employees in the establishments in which the employees usually report to work. As facility administrator, you must be aware of the various OSHA requirements and comply fully with them; harm to your employees and severe OSHA fines can result from noncompliance.

Employee Awareness

Employee education regarding established safety measures within the facility should begin with the employee's handbook issued at the time of hiring. Further and more specific instructions can be disseminated by periodic lectures and films, signs, and posters. (The National Safety Council provides excellent posters free of charge.)

An employee suggestion box placed in a well-traveled area of the facility could aid in establishing better safety policy. Employees should be encouraged to report violations, both structural and personal, and to suggest better safety strategy. Monthly awards might be instituted for the best safety suggestion received.

To further educate employees, the scientific application of color can identify high-risk areas requiring special caution. The following paint colors have been accepted nationally as safety standards:

1. *Soft green* is usually used for production machines because of its restfulness and general eye appeal.
2. *Cream* is used to define moving parts requiring manual supervision, since it relieves eyestrain.
3. *Bright red* is reserved for fire protection apparatus. Columns or rolls in which fire extinguishers or hoses are mounted should be banded with red high enough to be seen throughout the surrounding area.
4. *Green* usually designates safety equipment and first aid; therefore, all first-aid stations and dispensaries should be painted green. If the wall behind the first-aid cabinet is green, the cabinet should be painted white with a green cross.
5. *Black* and *yellow* should be used to create greater visibility of potentially dangerous objects. Hoists, cranes, elevator doors, and similar moving equipment, as well as low beams, stairways, pits, and door edges should be painted yellow with black bands. Traffic aisles are usually bordered by white or yellow strips a few inches wide to separate them from work and storage areas.
6. *Orange* also provides high visibility and should be used to warn workers of definite hazards. Machine guards around drives or hazardous machines, any dangerous vehicle, and the entire length, including uprights, of any conveyor or similar system, should be painted orange.
7. *Blue* designates electrical switch boxes and control panels, mounted on either walls or machines.

Generally speaking, large ducts should be painted the same as wall or ceiling areas, while pipelines can be painted identifying colors. The basic color standards for piping are:

red: fire protection
yellow or orange: dangerous materials
green, white, gray, aluminum: safety materials
bright blue: protection gases or liquids

Additional, more specific measures to educate employees in safety procedures will be covered in the section on fire prevention later in this chapter.

Safety Inspections

Safety inspections of the entire facility should be conducted on at least a weekly basis by the security department to uncover and report any and all unsafe conditions. Hazards that come about as a result of equipment deterioration, changes of the building proper, manner of merchandise stocking, and replacement of merchandise or personnel shall be subject to report.

THE EMERGENCY PREPAREDNESS PROGRAM

The emergency preparedness program must at all times be current, prepared for all emergencies that might arise, including disasters of any type that might present hazards to life and/or property. Here you must include fire; natural disasters such as hurricanes, tornadoes, earthquakes; and manmade disasters such as bomb threats and other acts of violence. The program must identify each possible disaster and explain how to recognize it; when it shall actually become a threat; and who is to do what, when, where, and how.

From the outset, all personnel must completely understand that any and all decisions regarding the emergency program shall come only from the director of security. Some people think that a separate fire marshal or chief should be assigned within the facility; I disagree. Since fire, safety, and overall security are the responsibilities of the security director, he should maintain single control so that all efforts in the above areas would be coordinated and inconsistencies in procedure kept minimal.

Policy Committees and Disaster Teams

Certain security professionals, I among them, feel that a special committee with direct representation of the security director should be established within the facility to draft *all* policy regarding *any* and *every* emergency. Others feel that each emergency calls for a specific committee. Both approaches include two levels of involvement: the committee(s) to draft policy and instruct procedure and the squad(s) to handle the actual emergency when it occurs.

Members of the emergency policy committee should come from all ranks of the facility personnel. Each should have some related knowledge and/or experience in the various potential emergency situations. In many business facilities, first aid is the only area of knowledge lacking fairly qualified emergency people. But this lack would obviously not occur in a hospital facility.

One of the greatest problems of any emergency program is to find *and keep* volunteers for the base teams. There are also problems in the training aspect of the program. Initial interest may be strong, but idealistic enthusiasm fades with the prospect of the discipline of long training. Add to this a normal personnel turnover problem, and you are faced with the possibility of no teams or only partial teams available at the time of an emergency. The paperwork required to keep your teams at an acceptable level is extremely important and should not be allowed to lapse. Another problem that should be avoided is that volunteers, despite their training in emergency situations, may be of little help when an emergency actually occurs. If they are overly idealistic or sensitive, they may panic or may not be able to maintain discipline in a crisis involving blood or real danger. Because they are professionals, the security staff of the facility should be leadership members of all disaster teams. Many of the problems of maintaining adequate volunteers can be overcome and the program enhanced only by giving the team members an incentive to join, train, stay, and perform.

I advocate that a disaster team be formed to handle each and every disaster that comes up as opposed to a separate team for each type of disaster. Since most hospital facilities are open 24 hours a day, three teams should be formed—one team for each 8-hour shift. The members of these teams would be fully trained to handle all emergencies and would receive additional compensation on an hourly basis to be added to their base wages. Pay for each training period would be time-and-a-half, the minimum paytime being one hour. Pay for each actual emergency would be double-time, the minimum paytime being one hour. Team personnel would be responsible to the director of security for all training and actual emergency service. The director of security would make the final decision as to who, in fact, would be a team member. Team personnel would be responsible for notifying the payroll department of the time spent on each training section and each actual emergency. The personnel department would have the responsibility of ensuring that the director of security was notified of any change in status of any member of the team. The members of each team would be fully trained in their teams' duties in every emergency situation. They would be trained to take care of any situation by themselves and would also receive leadership training to allow them to supervise the balance of the people in the facility who would answer all calls for help.

Equipment and Communication

In order for any emergency preparedness program to work, there must be a means of communicating all desired information to all involved personnel. Such communication must not cause panic of any kind. I suggest a three-way system of signals: a verbal announcement over the public address system in conjunction with a simultaneous series of colored lights and a system of clearly posted signs. The verbal announcement could consist of a series of numbers such as 111, 666, or 999. The accompanying flashing lights, such as green, yellow, red, would be placed at specified points throughout the facility; naturally, they would be placed in areas that are covered at all times, such as the nurses' station on each floor, and over each exit door of the facility. In addition to the flashing lights, directional arrows in corridor areas should indicate the fastest route to nearby exits. These arrows, preferably electrically operated and tied into the emergency lighting system, should be strobe-type high intensity lights, since normal lights cannot be seen through smoke.

To complete the emergency communication system, each facility telephone should be equipped with a decal giving a number to be called to report an emergency. I strongly advise that this number be the recognized 911 emergency number in use in most big cities. Your inhouse telephone system will have to be wired so that when the number is dialed, a special alarm will sound at the switchboard. The call would then receive top priority by your switchboard operator, who would take all necessary action as posted at the switchboard. Since all calls would be routed to the switchboard, it stands to reason that all calls for assistance would emanate from the switchboard, thus assuring that the entire emergency preparedness program could be started in motion from this point. Since the emergency control center would be at the main security desk, the onduty security chief would also automatically receive the emergency call in order to sound further alarms, and to proceed with the initial emergency steps during such times as the switchboard might be closed.

During regular hours, the switchboard operator would announce 111 in specified areas of the facility. Such coded announcement would alert only the members of the emergency and security teams on duty. Their arrival on the scene would dictate whether further announcements should be made. At the sounding of the initial call, security would get walkie-talkies to the scene of the emergency for further communication. In this way, the entire facility would not be aware of the potential danger, and panic would be avoided. Should the situation warrant it, emergency notification could be called and flashed to all areas, and the facility vacated. In this instance, the red light warning would be combined with audible alarms such as a bell or siren.

At all times, all personnel of the facility must be reminded that saving human life is paramount, and all personnel must be kept from seeing or hearing any signs of panic. Your failure to furnish the security section with the necessary tools and equipment to handle each potential emergency could cost lives as well as the facility itself. The exact type and amount of equipment required will depend largely upon the type and size of the facility being protected. However, basics would include items necessary for communications, such as phones, alarms, walkie-talkies, etc.; items necessary to fight fire, such as sprinklers, extinguishers, fire carts, etc.; and items necessary to contain and reduce damage, such as tarpaulins, bomb blankets, boarding materials, etc. Your director of security must prepare a master diagram of the facility to show the placement of all equipment, alarms, exits, and fire areas; this diagram must be posted at the security center from which instructions shall come.

General Employee Education

Everyone who has any access to the facility must be aware of emergency exits and procedures. The extent of such education shall, of course, differ according to the actual potential of each person's involvement in the emergency.

Education in emergency procedures, as in basic safety, should start with the employee's handbook. This handbook should, however, contain only the general information that is essential to allow the employee to react to the program. Unfortunately, you must protect the facility against those individuals who would actually create emergencies; do not provide enough information to make them totally aware of all protection and alarm systems, or they will construct an emergency by avoiding such detectionary devices. The handbook material can be further explained and additional information disseminated at departmental meetings and through signs and periodic drills.

As noted previously, small and yet easily seen paste-on signs giving the emergency telephone number should be attached to every telephone. In addition, such information should appear on 5" x 7" signs on every employee bulletin board and on every door leading out of every employee area. Near these signs, additional signs of approximately 11" x 14" should be posted to explain to all personnel their general duties upon hearing an emergency announcement. These signs must clearly and concisely identify each emergency recognition signal and the proper action to be taken. The signs must be made so as to stand out from surrounding areas. The function of all flashing light signals and electric directional arrows must be clearly labeled, and employees must receive adequate orientation, through the handbook and frequent drills.

The hospital administrator will have to make the decision whether or not to disrupt the facility by calling practice drills. Drills and evacuation cause not only disruption, but loss of time from assigned jobs. However, when an emergency occurs, it is obviously essential that the response be correct and efficient. The greatest advantage of frequent drills is that the correct behavior and procedures become rote and routine, eliminating much of the need for quick and independent thought and decision in an emergency, when panic might otherwise take over. Fire drill procedure is discussed in detail in the section on fire prevention, following.

Employee and patient complaints regarding drills and precautions can easily be dealt with by using signs which explain that any inconvenience is for the protection of the individual, or by explanatory sessions when advisable.

To summarize the emergency preparedness program, the best preparedness combines general personnel orientation, posted warnings and instructions, a trained corps of emergency workers, and periodic practice drills and program reassessments.

MEASURES FOR SPECIFIC EMERGENCIES

Fire

Fire is the most frequent of all major emergencies. Your emergency team must therefore be fully trained by a local fire department on all aspects of fire fighting and methods of fire prevention. Such training should be relatively extensive, not a mere overview; it will pay for itself if you are ever faced with a fire problem. The knowledge and training of your inhouse emergency team, led by your security department, will eventually save you many times the payroll cost of the training program. By obtaining this protection, you also will be conforming to OSHA requirements.

Every facility, regardless of size, must have a workable *and working* fire-prevention program. Management must recognize the program's importance by accepting and backing its policies and procedures, and by agreeing to enforce disciplinary measures against any and all violators. Conversely, a "bonus" type of reward for individuals and/or departments who show extra effort in aiding the program should be established and publicized. Without such managerial support, the program of fire prevention will grow lax and ultimately fail.

Each employee must be made aware of the following:

1. Safe methods of handling any hazards within the immediate work area.
2. Proper disposal methods of flammable wastes such as rags, paper, and combustible fluids.
3. The advantages of good housekeeping principles.
4. The importance of strict compliance with the rules concerning the facility's specific fire precautions.
5. Proper use of fire extinguishers.
6. The principles involved in the automatic sprinkler system. No obstructions must be placed in a way that may make the system inoperable or inefficient.
7. Locations and accompanying hazards of vulnerable fire areas.
8. Correct operation methods for all alarm systems.
9. Proper conduct in the event of fire.
10. Location of all fire equipment, exits, and evacuation routes.

In addition to the time set aside for drills, management must also set aside time, and provide monetary incentive, for the education of the fire team. In accord with acceptable security practices, the following must be taken into consideration:

1. The area of the premises to be covered
2. The nature of the fire hazards present in these areas
3. The time required for the local fire department to arrive

With the above needs defined, the number of fire teams must be established and the members of these teams drawn from every department of the facility. Each member must be assigned specific duties on the team, and must be trained as a team worker; everyone must understand that individual actions and unauthorized decisions are prohibited.

I believe that a total of two hours' training should enable all team members to learn their respective duties. Absolute team functioning can be established only through periodic drills, held on a weekly basis for at least the first six weeks after training and on a monthly basis thereafter. New members recruited to replace members no longer active would, of course, have to undergo the two hours of initial training.

Assuming that periodic fire drills involving all personnel have been approved by management, I will outline the basic drill procedure. The fire drill begins with a series of alarms to alert personnel. The actual alarm bell obviously must be loud and distinctive, sounded only in the event of fire drill or actual fire. If a series of alarms is used, all personnel must be fully educated as to the significance of each. For example:

Signal #1:   Cease work.
Signal #2:   Shut off machines, clear aisles.
Signal #3:   Line up.
Signal #4:   Move out.

Assigned fire wardens must assure that all drills are carried out smoothly and safely. They must also check for any personnel who either have not heard the alarm or are evacuating too slowly. All such individuals and situations should be identified and reported so that the security director/fire marshal can determine the cause of noncompliance; if it stems from a weakness in the system, it must be corrected, and if it stems from a lack of cooperation on the part of the involved personnel, it must be reported to the personnel department for further action in accordance with the enforcement policies of the program. To be effective, fire drills should be held at least monthly.

For the control and elimination of unnecessary fire hazards, I have developed a "motivation program" for facility-wide use, monitored by the security department. Under the plan, a security officer places a "reminder tag" at the point of a fire prevention violation and records the violation and the tagging in the security journal. If the department head of the violating area takes no actual action to remove the violation after a reasonable period of time, this is recorded in the security journal. The security director then issues to the department head a "motivation sheet" outlining the violation. The department head is required, within 24 hours, to report to his or her immediate superior, that superior's superior, and the security director what action has been taken to alleviate the situation. Again failing to respond, the department head is issued a "violation notice," copies of which are distributed to the head of the facility and the chairman of the board. This system ensures that the situation is corrected and helps you avoid OSHA fines, which usually run into thousands of dollars per offense per day.

The fire team's approach to fighting a fire should be similar to the approach to general disasters recommended previously. The fighting of a fire of any consequence would, of course, involve almost all of the members of the facility as well as the local fire department. When the fire department arrives, the members of the facility disaster team are usually relieved of responsibility, but their participation may be needed again for the clean-up operation.

Bomb Threat

Twenty years ago, the bomb threat did not appear in most emergency manuals. Today, many pages are devoted to it. However, almost all of the procedures boil down to waiting until the correct officials arrive and then following their advice. I do not feel that the entire facility should be placed on the edge of panic because a bomb threat has been received. In view of the sophisticated types of bombs presently available, I doubt the wisdom of conducting a bomb search. You generally will have no idea what the bomb looks like; it can be extremely small and impossible for amateur eyes to detect. (Letter bombs are obvious examples.) It is foolish to proceed on a search without the expertise of a trained bomb squad, however, you as the administrator must decide how much is to be done when a bomb threat is received. If there were a foolproof procedure, I would outline it here.

It is essential that all of the facts surrounding a bomb threat be recorded precisely. See Appendix A for a simple, self-explanatory form to be filled out by the person receiving the threat, usually the telephone operator. Attached to the form should be a clear guide to the procedures to be followed, as well as a checklist to record that each procedure was, in fact, followed. A supply of similar bomb threat reports must be kept readily available at the telephone switchboard as well as at the main security desk. The training of the telephone operator should include a course on how to keep calm and to elicit information while gathering essential identification about the caller. The operator must respond automatically. The following sign should be posted on the switchboard:

> Keep caller on the line as long as possible. Ask the caller to repeat message.
>
> Ask where bomb is. Ask what kind of bomb. Ask when it will go off.
>
> Advise caller the building is occupied and innocent people could get hurt.
>
> Give careful note to any background sounds such as motors, music, etc., that may give a clue as to the caller's location.

The sign should be printed with clear-cut letters; do not expect typewritten instructions to be followed in a crisis. In addition, the switchboard should be equipped so that the operator can press a button and automatically alert another person to pick up an extension and concentrate on identifying the caller's mannerisms, while at the same time recording the entire conversation. If possible, a third person could alert the telephone company to try to put a trace on the incoming call.

The facts of the call must then immediately be passed to the security director or the director's onduty senior representative. At this time the operator should also notify the fire and police officials. If the facility procedure calls for a bomb search to be conducted, a coded message should start the search at this point. If the security department has properly prepared in advance, the facility has been diagramed into preset areas. In each area, search areas should be listed on index cards stored at the central security desk; the cards should clearly state the specific cautions to be taken in each area, likely hiding spots in the area, and the most probable type and size of bomb. Upon receiving the call, all members of the emergency team should immediately go to their preassigned areas, collect the search cards, and start the search. If necessary, area personnel could assist. Immediately after the search of each area, the report of each area must be relayed to the main security desk. Further actions will be as directed by local officials who should, by now, have been summoned.

Preparation for bomb threats and actual explosions should include assuring adequate protection of classified documents, proprietary information, and other essential records. A well-planted, properly charged device could destroy records vital to your day-to-day operations.

Organize and train an evacuation unit consisting of key members of personnel; coordinate their training with that of other personnel so that evacuation procedures and leadership roles are known and respected. One consideration during a bomb threat is priority of evacuation. Always evacuate the floor levels on and above the danger area as quickly as possible. Training in this type of evacuation should be available from police, fire, or other knowledgeable units within the community. The evacuation unit should also be trained in search techniques, or you may prefer a separate search unit. To be proficient in searching the building, the unit members must be thoroughly familiar with all hallways, rest rooms, false ceilings, and every conceivable location in the building where an explosive or incendiary device might be concealed. It must be remembered that when the police or fire department arrive at the building, the contents and the floor plan will probably be unfamiliar to them. Thus, it is extremely important that the evacuation and search units be thoroughly trained and familiar with the floor plan as well as immediate outside areas.

The evacuation and search units should be trained only in evacuation and search techniques; they should not be expected to attempt to neutralize, remove, or have other contact with the device. If a strange or suspicious object is encountered, it should not be touched. Its location and description, as best as it can be provided, should be reported to the security director or other person designated to receive this information. If the danger zone is identified or located by the caller, the area should be blocked off or barricaded with a clear zone of 300 feet until the object has been removed or disarmed or danger has otherwise passed.

During the building search, a rapid two-way communication system is of utmost importance. Such a system can be readily established through the use of existing telephones. But the use of radios during a search can be dangerous. The radio could cause premature detonation of an electric initiator blasting cap.

The signal for evacuating the building in the event of a bomb threat should be the same as that used for evacuation in the event of fire. The use of different signals for bomb threats may create unnecessary panic and confusion.

If the building is evacuated, controls must be established immediately to prevent unauthorized access to the building. These controls may have to be provided by management. If proper coordination has been effected with the local police and other agencies, they may assist in establishing controls to prevent re-entry into the building until the danger has passed. The personnel must be removed to a safe distance from the building to protect them against debris and other flying objects in the event of an explosion. Once the building is evacuated, all electricity, gas, and fuel lines should be cut off at the main switch.

During the search, the medical personnel of the building should be alerted to stand by in the event of an explosion. Fire-brigade personnel should be alerted to stand by with fire extinguishers if necessary.

Pre-emergency plans should include a temporary facility relocation in case an explosion makes the building untenable for a considerable period of time. (See Appendix A, "Bomb Threats and Search Techniques," prepared by the U.S. Department of the Treasury, Bureau of Alcohol, Tobacco and Firearms.)

Riots and Civil Disorders

Here the major responsibilities for action rest with the local authorities; your involvement would consist mainly of reporting the facts and then following the authorities' instructions. For plate glass windows and doors, your emergency team, maintenance department, and security department should have precut, prenumbered plywood sheets which can be immediately and securely fastened from inside the building. These sheets are not intended to protect the glass, but to protect your employees and the area from flying glass, the elements, and the people involved in the disorder.

Your emergency squad's basic training should have covered all of the requirements necessary to control the disorder. (These training guidelines were outlined earlier in this chapter.) However, if you do not have an emergency team already trained and standing by, you should make on-the-spot provisions to ensure that the following rules be taken into consideration during civil disorders:

1. Do not threaten or attempt to bully those involved in the disorder. Bullying will not solve any portion of the problem; it could exacerbate it. Make sure that you can fully back up anything that you say; do not hesitate to back it up if necessary.
2. Do all that you can to persuade and reason with those involved to change their position. Turn the tide by turning their minds. Insert some ideas of common interest; speak to them as people rather than combatants.
3. Make sure that you remain calm and firm.
4. Where circumstances permit—and this is usually done by local officials—bring in someone of importance to talk to the people involved.
5. If the crowd becomes violent or irrational, do not allow your pride or frustration to diminish your own rationality. Keep out of the way, protect your employees, and rely on public officials to quell the violence and disperse the participants.

Strikes

Here you shall find yourself pitted against people you know, people with whom you associate daily, people who feel they have a legitimate and concrete dispute with what you as management represent. Force and verbal abuse will only create greater problems—immediately and after the strike has been settled. The chances are very good that your emergency team will, in this instance, be on the "other" side. Therefore, you will have to rely solely upon your security department to bring you through the problem period. But you must recognize that management and labor are apart and should stay apart until the negotiating team settles the strike.

Do not allow your security force to mix with or in any way confront the people on the picket line. Do not show any sign of force to the picketers. If your security force was not armed before the strike, do not arm them now. This is not to say that defensive weapons such as clubs should not be brought to areas where trouble might occur. If necessary, they should, but it is absolutely necessary to keep all such items completely out of sight.

Your security force should set up a command post from which all actions of the strikers can be observed and photographed. Each posted security officer or observer must be in immediate radio communication with the command post. There must be someone at the command post telephone at all times, preferably someone whose voice is known to all nonstriking personnel. The same voice should issue all orders which need to be issued by telephone. No one should be allowed to issue any orders or effect any movement of any type until it has been cleared and fully sanctioned by the post.

All reports of any type must be forwarded to the post and recorded in a special strike journal maintained at the post. All photographs should be taken by a professional photographer, who should maintain complete and accurate records; such records may be necessary in court at a later date.

In addition, the photographer should advise the journal clerk of each series of photographs taken. This information must be recorded in as much detail as necessary in the journal. Once the strike has been settled, all information concerning it should be filed away for future necessary reference. At no time should any part of the file be used for anything but strictly legitimate needs. After a strike is settled, everyone's state of mind is different than it was during the strike.

Chapter 6

Interdepartmental Coordination

Throughout previous chapters, I have stressed the imperative independence of the security department. Security should not be under the middle management control of the personnel department, but must report directly to the facility administrator or to a management-level director of security, who in turn reports directly to the facility administrator.

Because the function of the security department affects the overall operation and general safety of all departments and employees, interdepartmental coordination between security and other facility departments is definitely necessary. Therefore, periodic interdepartmental meetings should be held. In addition, facility management must carefully ensure that the director of security is promptly informed of any changes in policy and procedure—on both a facility-wide and an individual department basis—that might affect the security function in any way.

Because of their particular importance, the security functions of the receptionist and the personnel and maintenance departments will be outlined more fully in this chapter. (Coordination between security staff and company auditors was covered in Chapter 4.)

THE RECEPTIONIST

The receptionist holds a very responsible position, and must therefore be capable of handling any of several impromptu situations. Without appearing dictatorial, he or she must be levelheaded and firm with the people entering the facility. This person must be capable of snap decisions that could, if wrong, cost the facility many dollars in lawsuits. The receptionist must be able to handle personal problems brought in by disturbed people and to prevent theft by recognizing potential problems and monitoring rather than accusing. The responsibilities are numerous.

Because so much of the receptionist's time is taken up with matters of security, the receptionist should be an official member of the security section, answerable only to the director of security. Such an assignment not only makes sense, but also prevents a conflict of published orders.

In some smaller facilities, the receptionist/guard may actually represent the only "security" that the facility has. In such cases, this person must challenge everyone who enters the facility and many of those who leave the facility. A good security device is an employee entrance through which all employees are required to enter and leave.

In those facilities in which an employee entrance is not practical, the receptionist will have to be trained to deal with security problems created by employees—for example, the executive who wishes to take a computer or dictating machine home to complete an important project. If this is clearly against facility policy, the receptionist must be properly trained to enforce the policy and, naturally, must be confident of administrative support. The receptionist who decides to be lenient in such situations could be costing the employer thousands and even hundreds of thousands of dollars annually. In health care facilities, where a single small, portable item costs thousands of dollars, losses could easily reach the million-dollar mark. As an example, laboratory technicians can remove microscopes, portable centrifuges, and other expensive laboratory equipment either for their own use or possibly for illegal sale. Any person working in any area of the facility is capable of similar improper or illegal actions.

The receptionist must also be trained to remain calm and efficient in the midst of panic and must know how to summon the necessary help. If firefighters or police suddenly arrive at the facility, he or she must, of course, know what to do and whom to contact. The receptionist must also know how to calm the overwrought person who comes as a patient or who accompanies a severely ill or wounded patient.

None of these responsibilities can be successfully taught by merely outlining the problems and possible answers on a sheet of paper and giving it to the newly hired receptionist. Although such a sheet can certainly help as a reference, correct and acceptable reactions to various problems require a sense of duty and understanding that must be instilled by thorough training. This training should be a function of the security director, but could, where necessary, be handled by the director of personnel in coordination and consultation with the security department. In either case, it is extremely important that the receptionist be a capable asset to the overall security program of the facility.

THE PERSONNEL DEPARTMENT

Time and time again, I have written and talked of the business fallacy of placing the personnel department on the same level as the Almighty. In far too many companies, the personnel department is "in charge" of all other departments.

With too much power, the personnel director can create serious problems. Where direct control of another department cannot be secured because of a strong department head, the personnel director might revert to calculated tricks to gain control. The department's personnel requests may be ignored, or people assigned who prove inadequate to the job descriptions submitted.

Other abuses of the personnel director that I have uncovered include the use of facility employees for personal jobs. Carpenters build garages, closets, etc., in the home of the personnel director, and facility management pays for the labor and materials. Dishonest personnel directors can run ghost payrolls; they can also methodically steal from retirement funds, profit-sharing funds, etc. Such cases are not often reported publicly because of the company's obvious embarrassment at having hired and given such autonomy to a dishonest executive. Thus, the apprehended dishonest personnel director is quietly terminated and placed out on the market to become someone else's problem.

Obviously, there are capable and honest personnel directors; my point is only that the company should never allow this individual unlimited and unchecked authority. And, as pointed out in Chapter 4, the personnel department must be included in facility-wide security audits.

If one would stop and review the responsibilities of the personnel department, one would easily see that many of their actions demand coordination with the security department. For example, all new employees and any employees being considered for promotion should be fully checked by the security department. This aspect of interdepartmental coordination between the security and personnel departments is also covered more fully in Chapter 4.

The security department must not be under the complete control of the personnel department. It is imperative that security be managed by a director of security answerable only to the chief executive of the facility. Periodic interdepartmental meetings are mandatory, led by a facility management representative, to maintain and improve lines of communication and cooperation. But the security department must remain independent of middle management control in order to retain its auditing objectivity and its singularity of function.

THE MAINTENANCE DEPARTMENT

For some unknown reason, one of the most trusted individuals of any facility is the maintenance supervisor. Maintenance workers are not, however, more trustworthy by nature than other employees. Yet the maintenance worker, by virtue of the job, requires almost unlimited access to the entire facility.

Under no circumstances should the maintenance staff have *carte blanche* to come and go as they please, or be issued master keys that would provide unnecessary access to high-risk areas. I do not intend that the maintenance department be needlessly restricted; but they must be held accountable, and since any area in which they work will be vulnerable to accident, theft, or fire, they must be placed under the jurisdiction and control of the security department. If this is not feasible, the facility administrator must call for absolute coordination between the two departments. I emphasize coordination. Any maintenance function that requires any change in the facility structure must be coordinated with security. As an example, the most effective key control system in the world is useless if the maintenance department changes a lock without informing the security department.

PART III

Responsibilities of the Security Staff

Chapter 7

Investigations and Report Writing

In earlier chapters, I have outlined the investigatory procedures involved in the full security check on entering, promoting, and terminating employees. Additionally, I have emphasized the importance of continual surveillance and periodic investigation as effective watchdogs of the facility internal controls program. To review these facets of security investigation, see Chapters 3 and 4.

INVESTIGATIONS—ACCIDENTS AND DISASTERS

All accidents and disasters must also be fully investigated by a qualified investigator to ascertain direct cause and determine the conditions that led to its happening. Every minor accident will not always warrant an intensive and detailed investigation, but the facts concerning every accident, regardless of how minor it appears to be, must be recorded. Major injuries would, of course, require full investigation. The decision as to what should and should not be investigated must be left to the discretion of the director of security or safety director.

Some security authorities suggest that any member of management or immediate supervisory staff can conduct the investigation. However, it is essential that the person be thoroughly trained in investigatory procedure. Members of management should contribute their knowledge of the accident and/or a preliminary report of the accident, but the official accident investigation should be left to a trained investigator who can be trusted to obtain all of the essential facts. Due to potential litigation involving management's liability in an on-premises accident, most facility attorneys will agree that a comprehensive investigative report at the time of the accident is mandatory.

The majority of the security department's investigations will concern claims against the facility. These claims will, of course, be presented under the provisions of civil law rather than criminal law. It is therefore imperative that the individual assigned to conduct facility investigations have a thorough knowledge of civil law; comprehensive knowledge of criminal law will not suffice, since the requirements of proof in one do not automatically apply to the requirements of proof in the other. It is essential that the investigator be aware of the terms and definitions of civil law — for example, the civil law defintion of "negligence," the different types, what in fact constitutes it, and how to apply the relative rules.

The investigator must be dedicated and thorough. Naturally, the investigator must be absolutely certain that all of the information recorded is factual. Too many "investigators" hired to gather factual background material go out and gather immediate reactions to a situation, accept these reactions as facts, and then create a mythical version of the situation, reporting opinion rather than fact. Such amateur investigations not only end up costing management money in the form of an additional investigation needed to separate fact from myth, but also make the facility vulnerable to a lawsuit.

It is equally essential that attorneys handling any defense of the facility be fully aware of all relevant facts. Using shortcuts or amateur techniques, too many investigators misapply the information they gather; sometimes they even discard evidence that does not support their theories of what happened. Obviously, the facility's attorneys must be assured that the information they get from the facility investigator is thoroughly researched and substantiated fact. Any areas of the investigator's report that present conflicting evidence or that appear sketchy or not fully substantiated should be questioned immediately. It is conceivable that a case, although investigated immediately after the situation occurred, may not come to trial for two or three years. While reviewing the report in preparation for a court appearance, the attorney might discover minor inconsistencies in the facts or the existence of information that may be judged speculative; with the passage of time, the investigator might not be able to explain the inconsistencies or easily relocate witnesses to resume interrogation.

The investigative report must indicate the source of all information. Again, the quality of your investigator is extremely important. Too many "investigators" have no idea what constitutes good or bad information. If, for example, the opposing attorneys can prove that a statement was taken from a person of questionable motivation or one prone to elaboration or exaggeration, obvious embarrassment and legal problems will ensue, to say nothing of the thwarting of justice. Therefore, each potential witness must be carefully considered. Is the individual credible? Was the individual physically positioned so as to be able to have witnessed what he or she claims? Once the witness is established as qualified, all statements must be

written down carefully in the individual's own words and signed by the witness. The investigator's report should then be prefaced by any necessary qualifying remarks concerning the credibility of the witness's statements. The attorney can then determine whether or not the information is usable and whether or not the witness will appear in court.

Another thing that must be taken into consideration is how the physical evidence should be retained for further use at a later date. It is not always possible to retain the physical evidence concerning an accident or other incident under investigation. For this reason, we must resort to diagrams and photographs. Obviously, it is essential that the diagrams or photographs truly reflect the area in question as it appeared at the time of the incident.

Naturally, if not capable of taking adequate photographs, the investigator should not hesitate to obtain the services of a qualified professional photographer. But it is essential that the photographer be made aware (from the investigator's standpoint) of how to reproduce the scene so that all factors pertinent to the situation under investigation are shown.

Careless investigation and inadequate photographs can lead to problems, as a recent case shows. A woman tripped on a piece of metal that was protruding from the ground in a public parking lot. Investigation disclosed that the piece of metal was a hook used to hold down a hockey net used by boys playing in the lot over the weekend. Because the owners of the property knew that the boys played hockey in the lot, the owners were responsible for making sure that such use did not make the lot unsafe for customers. Their failure to locate and remove the hook could be determined sufficient negligence to allow the woman to sustain a claim for damanges. The subsequent investigation was not conducted efficiently. No diagram of any type was made to illustrate the appearance, size, or location of the hook. The photographs were terrible; the position of the sun and of the photographer produced a fine photograph of a man's shadow. And to compound inefficiency, the hook was removed from the ground by the investigator after he took the photographs; additional photographs could therefore not be taken, and there were no witnesses with him to testify as to the height and appearance of the hook in its original position. The final investigative report consisted of one paragraph. No effort was made to determine if there were any witnesses, if anything had been done, or if anything should have been done. The photographs were attached to the report and forwarded to the home office of the investigative agency, arriving approximately one week after the accident. The woman sustained rather heavy injuries and a lawsuit will almost certainly result.

If this investigator had been truly qualified and trained, he would have covered all of the area involved. He would have made sure that the location of the hook was shown by diagram as well as reports and photographs, and

he would have carefully recorded by photograph the height of the hook in such a manner that it could easily be determined whether or not it clearly constituted a hazard.

This same set of circumstances applies to all cases under investigation. At the time of the accident, it is very easy to determine what did occur and how. However, a week or two after the accident, it becomes almost impossible to recreate the situation with total accuracy. At the accident scene, should it be necessary to remove evidence immediately in order to allow traffic to pass through the area, the investigator should mark the area with chalk or similar means in order to preserve as much data as possible. In the event of a death or other serious incident, the investigator must not move *anything* until such time as all pertinent data have been recorded and the authorities say that free access into the area can safely resume. If a thorough investigation dictates that traffic must be rerouted around the incident site, the investigator must seek some traffic control assistance. If it is not possible to reroute traffic, the investigator must work as quickly as possible; however, speed should not affect thoroughness, since the investigation is obviously more important than traffic flow.

To prepare diagrams, it is not necessary that the investigator be an artist. All that is necessary is the accurate recording of the distances between pertinent objects. The actual placement within the accident scene can then be recorded by an artist using accurate sketches. The investigator unable to draw diagrams may have to go into far more detail in order to present a comprehensive set of facts to the artist preparing the final copy.

It is of ultimate importance that the investigator be aware of personal limitations and be truthful about such limitations. If unable to draw a diagram or take a photograph, the investigator must be willing to admit this and to seek outside help. If unable to determine good information from bad information, or unable to record the facts without attempting to shade them to fit theories, the investigator should be replaced. It is the responsibility of the director of security to ensure that the items in question are reported as they should be reported, and that the assigned investigator is knowledgeable.

I cannot overemphasize the importance of a thorough, professional investigation. Failure to follow high investigative standards can cost a lot of money in wasted effort, potential lawsuits, and inflated insurance claims. Of course, high insurance claims will ultimately be reflected in the facility's future premiums, provided, obviously, that the insurance carrier agrees to renew the policy.

If your facility does not have a large enough security staff to include capable full-time investigators, you should hire an outside detective agency to perform the necessary investigations. But not just anyone, insurance-

trained or not, is capable of investigative work. Knowledge of proper investigative techniques, as well as skill in interrogation, are absolutely essential in obtaining all the information necessary to prove an insurance claim and/or obtain a favorable trial outcome and settlement.

REPORT WRITING

The most important element of any investigation is the report. A brilliant investigator can conduct an extremely thorough investigation and then render it worthless by submitting an inadequate report. I will not attempt here to give a course on report writing; however, I will outline what a good report should contain so that you know what to demand.

The report is both an instrument for transmitting to facility management immediate information about what in fact transpired and an instrument of factual record to be submitted later to authorities, insurance companies, or facility attorneys. The report takes several forms and is used for various reasons. You shall be faced primarily with the format and the narrative report. For the most part, the routine of security will be handled by the format report, so this form will be what you see most often. However, more involved situations will call for the narrative report, in which the who, what, where, when, why and how questions will be answered.

Regardless of type, the report will obviously suffer if it is handled by someone who cannot put into words exactly what happened. You should never allow or accept the submission of rewritten reports, especially from an outside agency, but should demand that your security consultant ensure that everyone assigned to security be trained in the writing of reports.

The *format report* will answer questions by a simple "yes" or "no," providing an overview of the daily status of the facility.

Dietary Department	Yes	No
Doors locked		
Stoves off		
Lights off		
Area free of hazards		
(etc.)		

If the security officer making the report finds conditions at the site that require action or further comment in the report, a brief narrative will be added to the printed format sheets.

The much more detailed *narrative report* will encompass the following:

1. Who: Full identification of all individuals involved in any way. Identification must include full names and addresses and specify degree of involvement.

2. What: Precise details about what happened, in sequential order, with all extenuating circumstances.

3. When: Exact time of *each* of the sequential events involved in the investigated incident. Times should be recorded to the second, if possible.

4. Where: Exact location of the incident and the placement of all involved individuals, objects, and possible witnesses.

5. How: Factual restructuring of the combination of causal agents effecting the occurrence of the incident. This must not be confused with *why*, which follows. The *how* is concerned with reasons; the *why* tends to involve excuses. In fulfilling the requirements of the *how* section, the investigator must explain how each involved participant or condition came into the picture and how his/her/its existence in the picture effected the end result. It is imperative that this area involve *only facts*; should any part involve any degree of conjecture, such must be clearly indicated.

6. Why: Full statements of all involved individuals, including passive witnesses, and carefully researched conjectures, identified as such, of the investigator. The majority of the "reasons" offered by those involved will tend to be excuses; it is the job of the investigator to differentiate between reasons and excuses. If people deemed "knowledgeable" declare that their versions of the events are totally factual, a competent investigator will still continue to dig further, and will present their words as only their opinions, qualifying all statements as necessary. Too many "investigators" merely parrot what has been told to them and record such material as facts.

Every item recorded in a report must be authenticated and qualified. Authentication is accomplished through photographs, copies of official records, diagrams, signed and/or witnessed statements, certificates, etc. Qualification of statements is clearly indicated by citing the source, as in

"John Doe stated...," and by full details of the witness's credibility (ulterior motive, physical state, physical position in relation to the incident, etc.).

The report itself, whether format or narrative, must be brief and to the point. Reports should be submitted only when absolutely necessary; too much paperwork can create confusion and sloppy work. A review of reports being submitted usually reveals that a few forms could be upgraded and integrated and a few could be deleted. Many otherwise good security directors attempt to solve new problems by instituting new report forms designed to cover once-in-a-lifetime occurrences. This obviously is not practical; the report form should be flexible enough to be usable for several occurrences, and the security officers should not have to seek out and become familiar with a wide variety of forms in order to prepare a potentially crucial report.

The professional security survey (see Chapter 2) should enumerate all of the incidents—disaster, safety, and overall security—that could conceivably happen in the facility, and suggest the number and type of format reports necessary to cover each situation. A hurricane, striking for the first time in fifty years, should not result in a new form entitled "The Hourly Hurricane Watch Report." Neither should there be reports to report on reports; format reports are certainly necessary, but they can and must be kept to a minimum.

Every security department should maintain a daily journal as part of its standard report-writing function. Located at a central post and available for scrutiny to only a select few, the daily journal would capsulize all events of each day. Each security officer on duty would submit entries to the journal regarding any *nonroutine* events. The journal keeps the need for report forms to a minimum, allows authorized people up-to-the-minute access to all pertinent information, keeps administrative costs down, and provides a central report location to monitor not only what has happened, but what has been done about it. There is only one report to view, and not a dozen. It is probable that many facilities would require still additional forms to cover major incidents; however, use of the journal does away with the costly and time-consuming practice of individual reports by each shift officer. As an example, if a facility has sixteen officers on each of three shifts, the security clerk is filing 336 preprinted format report forms a week, representing a terrific waste of time, equipment, stock, and money. (Discussion of a separate security journal, to be created during an on-premises labor strike, appears in Chapter 5.)

Chapter 8

Apprehensions and Interrogations

There are, of course, many laws protecting the rights of the individual confronted or apprehended as a criminal suspect. One can open a whole Pandora's box when one stops the forward motion of another individual. Unlawful apprehension methods should never arise, and will not arise if your security force knows what it is doing.

Apprehension of a suspect appears to be warranted when a person is *known* to be removing an item that is *known* to belong to someone else or is *known* to be in an area without having authorized access. In either case the confronting individual must have the authority to intercede the situation. When everything falls into place, the confronting individual must proceed with extreme caution in order to act within the civil laws protecting the accused.

An apprehension must never take place merely on the word of another individual. If you do not witness the purported crime, or do not have corroborating testimony from an extremely credible witness, do not act. Remember that a suspect must be assumed innocent until guilt can be proved absolutely. Improper accusation and treatment of the suspected individual, employed or not employed, can be infinitely more costly than the losses sustained by the actual crime.

When dealing with your own employee as suspect, you have more latitude because apprehension can be put off until such time as certainty of guilt does exist or you decide that an interview with the suspect is warranted. The seriousness of the offending act usually dictates what action must be taken and how it should be taken. Again, a well-trained security force can serve you well in the determination of the proper approach.

An interview with an offending employee will often not only straighten out the "offense," but also allow you to keep a good, albeit misdirected, employee on your staff. I could recount hundreds of examples in which such actions saved a good employee who years later became an extremely

valuable asset to the employer. Interviews also have a way of revealing information that leads to the uncovering of wholesale theft or similar types of
group criminal activities. Sometimes information gained in an interview
allows you to take action and avert potential problems involving union
workers and/or general employee morale.

Not every employee who steals should be apprehended and prosecuted
"to the fullest extent of the law." Each case must be handled on its individual merits. This is not say that dishonesty should be condoned; obviously it must be stopped. However, *action* and not *reaction* is the
necessary course.

Regardless of which procedure you use to detect and apprehend the
dishonest employee, you must eventually get to the point of interrogation.
If the interrogating officer is not a professional, and either fails to elicit
complete and factual information from the "suspect," or attempts to elicit
information through unlawful force or other methods involving a threat to
the individual's civil liberties, the entire investigation and apprehension
will be worthless.

There are several advocates of the polygraph (lie detector) as an aid to
the interrogating process. Very few people who use polygraph machines
are really qualified as experts. It is a machine that can be easily abused.
And since it is only a machine, it should never be trusted to produce absolute, credible fact. The truly professional polygraph expert uses the
machine only for what it is, a tool *to aid* in interrogation, capable of revealing only indications of behavior, which must then be interpreted precisely
by thoroughly trained behavioral experts. The polygraph should never be
used whimsically; this will constitute abuse of the civil rights of the supsect,
who could, consequently, be set free.

In all cases involving apprehension and interrogation, seek the help of a
professional. If truly professional, your director of security will conscien-
tiously seek the help of the local, state, and federal police when help is
needed.

Chapter 9

The Security Instruction Manual

Whether directed to the security personnel specifically or to other personnel of the facility, security instructions must be in writing and must be easily understood. The instructions for the security personnel should be issued in manual form, and any additions or deletions should be made on a per-page basis, so that the entire page is replaced when revised. At times, this will necessitate addendum pages. As an example, assume that the initial instructions appear on page 3, but subsequently a correction is necessary on page 3 that runs over into what would ordinarily be page 4. To avoid the necessity of retyping and rearranging the entire section of the manual to accommodate the revision, the additional material can be placed on an additional following page, designated as 3-A.

The following material represents a complete set of general security instructions used as part of a facility security program which I oversaw. I suggest that the reader use the information as a basic outline, copying the relevant information and making changes where necessary. Specific instructions regarding individual patrol and post responsibilities are discussed in Chapter 10.

SECURITY SECTION INSTRUCTIONS

The instructions contained herein nullify all previously issued instructions, including shift orders bearing dates previous to above.

All security officers are reminded that they are charged with the responsibility of safeguarding the assets of this company, and that no other section or individual is so charged or has the privileges of performing duties to that end. Therefore, you have been specially selected; your total performance is the only measure by which we may determine if such a selection was a proper one or not. You are a direct representative of this company, and your appearance in the eyes of all involved individuals— executives, employees, and visitors—could be the basis upon which our company is judged. For these reasons, it is imperative that each of you fully understand and follow the instructions contained herein.

(The special orders that come about from time to time should be issued to the security personnel in the form of numbered shift orders so that each order has its own sheet of paper and is easily identified. At a later date, the shift orders that have become outmoded can be, by another shift order, cancelled and thereby removed from the security officer's file. The shift orders that have reached the stage of permanent instructions can then be recapped and replaced in the security instructions booklet, at which time all reference by shift order would be made through the instruction manual.)

The purpose of this manual is to outline the policies and procedures that must be followed by all personnel who are assigned duty with the home-office security section. Each person is charged the responsibility of knowing and following all of the policies and procedures in this manual. The sergeant of each shift is charged with the responsibility of ensuring that each security member on the shift is fully aware of the contents of this manual and follows all instructions.

Responsibility

The home-office security section is charged with the responsibility of safeguarding the assets of the company against loss through any means. This responsibility *does not* confer disciplinary or enforcement powers on the security section or any member thereof. The security section is not a law-enforcement section; it is not an enforcement body of any kind. It will perform its assigned tasks by reporting all violations of the company's policies and/or procedures through the channels outlined herein.

Organization

The following organizational regulations and job descriptions will be adhered to until further notice.

Supervisor

The supervisor is responsible to management for the efficient organization and operation of all matters of security pertaining to the home-office security section, which encompasses the home office and distribution centers of this company. This responsibility is to include all matters pertaining to personnel, operations planning, and training of the security section. The supervisor will be assisted in this assignment by the shift sergeant.

Shift Sergeant

The shift sergeant is responsible only to the supervisor of the home office and distribution center security section, and will obey only those orders received through this source. The responsibility of this position includes complete control of the assigned shift, and encompasses supervision over training, scheduling, and all aspects of the security policies and/or procedures in effect at the time of assignment. The shift sergeant will ensure that each security member on the shift is fully aware of each of the standing shift orders. He or she will be responsible for efficient and immediate follow-up of each incident that occurs during the shift and will make recommendations, based on the incidents the shift experiences, regarding any changes in security policies and/or procedures that might possibly benefit the company. The shift sergeant is in complete charge of the shift and has complete authority over all security officers assigned to the shift. They will take their orders only from their sergeant. Other responsibilities of this position include raising and lowering the flag, seeing that parking and package control regulations are adhered to, and preparing and submitting the designated format report at the end of each shift.

Security Officers

Uniform and Apprearance. At all times, security officers shall report for duty in neat and clean prescribed uniforms. The appearance of security officers is an indication of their attitude; therefore, they must be neatly groomed at all times while on duty. The prescribed uniform will always be worn on duty and, except for published changes, will be considered complete as prescribed. Officers must wear the hat and breast badges in full view at all times while on duty and *never* while not on duty. At no time are security officers allowed to "flash their badges," and violation of this rule will be grounds for immediate dismissal.

Attitude and Demeanor. Diplomacy in every circumstance will reflect our position and will enhance the position of our section. A "police" attitude *will not be tolerated.* Consideration and respect for others must be the watchword of the security officer at all times and all circumstances.

Smoking. Smoking, in moderation and in such a manner as to reflect credit on our section, is allowed on any post situated in an area where smoking is normally allowed. Good manners should naturally govern the use of this privilege. Officers must be aware of the obvious fire hazards that accompany smoking and must not create any such hazards.

Coffee and Lunch Breaks. All such breaks will be governed by the shift sergeant and should be taken only when a suitable replacement is available to cover the post. At no time may an officer leave the post without proper permission and replacement. If an emergency occurs that requires the officer to leave the post, the officer shall first call the shift sergeant or, in the event of "personal emergencies," post #1, and explain the situation at hand. The security officer will receive a coffee break of ten minutes, both in the morning and in the afternoon. The lunch break for personnel on the 0800 to 1600 shift will be thirty minutes, and will be governed by the same instructions. All lunch and coffee breaks are subject to postponement if the situation so warrants.

Fraternization. Any social contact with personnel employed by this company and/or its affiliates and personnel arriving at the facility for business reasons *will not be tolerated.* Failure to abide by this rule will result in dismissal. Security officers must not, either by word or action, become involved in any relationship that might indicate guilt of fraternization. This rule will be strictly enforced.

Conversation. All discussions by a security officer will be carried out in a conversational tone, without any attitude or tone that might imply rudeness, a braggartly manner, or a feeling of superiority. All personnel, regardless of position, should be addressed as "sir" or "ma'am." All answers to questions will be as complete as possible. If the officer's knowledge or orders prohibit a full answer, all questions must be referred to the immediate supervisor. At all times when answering the telephone, the officer must identify post, location, and self; this information will be followed by "May I help you?"

Newspaper Releases. At no time and under no circumstances should a security officer reveal any information to a member of the press. All such releases are the responsibility of supervisory personnel, and any questions from media representatives, including newspaper, magazine, radio, and television personnel, should be referred to the security officer's supervisor.

Absenteeism and Tardiness. Any unnecessary absenteeism and/or tardiness will not be tolerated. The security officer who needs to request a day off must call in and notify the shift sergeant, allowing enough time for the shift sergeant to find acceptable temporary coverage. Tardiness must be handled similarly. Prolonged absenteeism will be accepted as the individual's method of submitting a resignation.

Laxness/Inability to Perform. Laxness and/or the inability to fulfill responsibility will be basis for dismissal. However, such dismassal shall occur only after the sergeant's report shows that the officer has been warned, but the inferior performance continues.

Adherence. The security officer, more than any other employee of this company, must adhere to every company policy and procedure. It is therefore imperative that each officer be fully aware of all such policies; failure to abide by them will be basis for immediate dismissal.

Reporting Time. All shift sergeants are expected to report for duty at least fifteen minutes prior to their scheduled time; all security officers are expected to report at least five minutes prior to their scheduled time.

Duties Scheduling. Post assignments will be on a weekly basis; all officers will be expected to perform the duties of the post to which they are assigned for each week. Weekly scheduling is intended to give the officers sufficient exposure to all security facets ultimately to enable each officer to perform each facility security task efficiently. By temporarily covering for other officers on their coffee and lunch breaks every day, each officer will receive training on the various posts assigned to this section. This should be done in the following manner: have the roving officer at the overhead doors post, sending the relieved officer to the next receiving post, sending that officer on in the same forward progression until the final post in the section is covered by the roving officer, who sends the last relieved officer on break. After break, this officer will report to the overhead doors post, thus beginning the cycle again. All personnel will, therefore, in the course of taking their prescribed breaks, relieve and cover all security posts in the section.

After-duty Hours. During hours when the facility is not normally open for business, the security officer must make note of all that occurs. This includes the opening of any doors not normally opened during these hours, the setting off of any alarms, the arrival of visitors, the delivery of merchandise, the removal of any facility property, the tardiness of relief officers, etc. Some of the above specific incidents have prescribed report forms on which to log the details; if specific forms do not exist, the information must be recorded in the security officer's regular shift report.

Patrol. In addition to the items specified for security check on the officer's log sheets for each facility area, the officer must be generally aware of situations requiring action. For example, the security officer is responsible for checking each office and public area to ensure that no electric lights, fixtures, or equipment have been left running. Public areas include corridors, rest rooms, etc. This patrol responsibility pertains to day as well as evening hours.

Emergency Procedures. In the course of the patrol, the security officer must be alert for any and all signs of fire, safety, or security hazards and must be prepared to take immediate and appropriate action, and then notify the following persons in the order listed:

(List of emergency personnel)

Other emergency numbers are posted on the red emergency board at the main desk. In case of power failure, the security officer must contact:

(Person so authorized)

Instructions to Officers. All security personnel are reminded that only the shift sergeant and/or security supervisors can issue orders to security personnel. All other personnel attempting to give orders to the security officer are to be advised, in a diplomatic manner, that the security officer cannot accept such orders and that they must contact either the shift sergeant or the supervisor to effect any changes. Security officers must not hesitate to follow this course of action; responsible executives will understand and comply. These instructions are clearly posted over each post; if someone other than the shift sergeant and/or the security supervisor approaches an officer with a request for an order change, the officer should refer the individual to the posted regulation.

Time Cards. All security personnel will show four punches per day on their time cards. These will represent time on duty, time out to lunch, time back from lunch, and time off duty. All security officers must sign their time cards. No person other than the section supervisor may write in any times on any time card.

Dry Cleaning. Every Tuesday, each officer must bring in at least two shirts, two pairs of trousers, and one jacket for dry cleaning. These items will be returned on the following Wednesday, and must be removed immediately from the security office. Each officer will list the clothing brought in for cleaning on a form that is posted on the bulletin board of the security office. Claims of lost articles will be honored only from this form.

Relief from Post. Security officers shall not leave a post for any reason, unless they are personally relieved by other officers or the shift sergeant. Officers should never leave their posts to answer telephone calls or paging announcements.

Mail and Merchandise Handling. No security officer shall, except for the purpose of saving lives or preventing property from being damaged or causing injury, handle any piece of mail or any parcel or carton in the distribution center or office area of the facilities. Mail and parcels received during hours when mail department personnel are not on duty may be accepted by security, but will be kept by the security personnel until an authorized member of the mail department arrives.

Standing Orders

Smoking. No smoking is allowed within the confines of the distribution centers, and each security officer will be alert for any violations or indications of violation of this policy. Violators will be reported to the supervisor of the area in which the violation occurs, to the security officer, and to the security officer's supervisor.

Traffic Regulations. See the special memo. (A memo updating standing orders on facility traffic and parking regulations was circulated to all security officers.)

ADT Alarms. Attached hereto is a chart showing the ADT alarm location, coverage, and functioning times. Each security officer shall study this chart.

Shift Orders. From time to time, new orders and changes in standing orders will be published via the shift orders. These will be issued as the situation demands and take effect as posted. All security officers must check the shift book each day as they report for duty. No excuses will be accepted for failure to comply with this order, and shift sergeants will be held solely responsible for ensuring compliance.

Acceptance of Valuables. No security officer should accept for safekeeping any money or merchandise. This includes checks, money orders, etc. Any person wishing to leave valuables with the security officer should be advised to contact this office first. This order is intended to cover valuables only.

Lost and Found. All articles should be reported via the lost and found reports. Security should not return any article to any person without that person's signature. All lost and found articles will be tagged (upper portion of tag to go on object, lower portion of tag to be attached to the report) and turned in at the security office at the end of the shift during which it was found.

Flag and Fringe Lights. The shift sergeant is responsible for ensuring that the flag storm (during bad weather) and garrison (during good weather) is raised at official sunrise and taken down at official sunset. The sergeant is further responsible for ensuring that the fringe lights, located in the executive board room, are lit at sunset and turned off at sunrise.

Chapter 10

The Security Guard: Posts and Patrols

In addition to the general instructions provided to each security employee in the instruction manual outlined in Chapter 9, specific duty instructions must be printed up and explained to each incoming officer.

LOCATIONS AND DUTIES OF POSTS

In a separate portion of the instruction manual, or in a looseleaf folder facilitating updates, all posts and their specific duties must be outlined. These post instructions should be printed on a page-per-post basis, and each individual page should be given to guards prior to their initial post assignments so that they can be fully aware of the relevant responsibilities and question any duties that are unclear before actually being on duty. A copy of the individual post orders should be attached to a clipboard and kept at the post, being passed from the guard on duty to the guard who relieves at the end of the shift or at lunch or coffee break. The security officer on duty at the post at the time the post is closed for the day will return the clipboard to the security office. The first security officer assigned to the post the next day will then pick up the orders before reporting to the post. Any changes in the standing orders will be attached to the clipboard.

The following represents a sample set of post orders used in a facility security program for which I was responsible. Immediately following the orders are a time conversion chart and sample memoranda showing changes in the standing orders.

OUTLINE
I. GENERAL INSTRUCTIONS

    a.   Beginning Shifts
    b.   Log

c. Tours
d. Emergency Calls
d. Emergency Calls
e. Strangers (See also Memorandum Re: Armed Guards.)
f. Vacating Post
g. Ending Shifts
h. Miscellaneous Questions

II. SPECIAL INSTRUCTIONS

a. Alarms
b. EKG Room
c. Laundry
d. Loading Platform Door (Receiving Dock)
e. Mailroom
f. Maintenance Stockroom (Emergency Supplies)
g. Rubbish Packer
h. Storeroom (Emergency Supplies)
i. Switchboard
j. Fire
k. Disaster

III. WALKING PATROL

a. Monday-Friday
b. Saturdays, Sundays and Holidays
c. Exterior Door Locking Schedule
d. Interior Door Locking Schedule
e. Exterior Door Unlocking Schedule
f. Interior Door Unlocking Schedule
g. Keys
h. Watchman's Clock Stations

IV. "STATIC" POSTS

a. Main Entrance Post
b. Nurses' Hall Guard

V. TIME CONVERSION TABLE

VI. MEMORANDA

GENERAL INSTRUCTIONS

MAXIMUM SECURITY IS ACHIEVED WHEN GUARDS ARE AT DIFFERENT LOCA-
TIONS IN THE HOSPITAL. OVERALL SECURITY IS EFFECTIVELY HALVED
WHEN GUARDS ARE PATROLLING SIDE BY SIDE.

BEGINNING SHIFTS

1. At the beginning of *every* shift, each guard punches in on the time clock located in the hall near the maintenance shop. There are two cards lableled for each shift. Each guard signs the time card beside the time punched by the clock.
2. At the beginning of the 1600-2400 hour (weekday) shift, two guards report to the maintenance shop for any special instructions, their log books, walkie-talkies, and keys.
3. At 0001, 0800, and (weekend) 1600 hours, the guards' logs from the previous shift are signed at the bottom with indication that walkie-talkie, keys, and any necessary special instructions were transferred.
4. All guards fill in the heading of their own logsheets (trainees do not fill in logsheets).
5. The schedule for use of the lecture hall and the auditorium should be checked at the beginning of each shift.

LOGS

1. Each guard should carry a log or a small notebook at all times for temporary notes, which should be transcribed onto log sheets before the end of the shift.
2. All unusual situations *must* be noted in the log with as much information as possible (e.g., trash accumulations, broken windows, etc.).
3. All significant incidents such as strangers, thefts, accidents, and/or injuries should be noted with as much information as possible.
4. If a trainee's name appears on a log sheet, a note (in parentheses) stating that the person is in training should follow.

TOURS

1. Each shift of eight hours (two guards) shall make at least three complete watchclock tours and three random tours of the complete hospital (except during hours of nurses' hall post).
2. During the hours of the nurses' hall post, random tours should be made by the walking guard as often as possible, as well as three complete watchclock tours.

3. For the sake of variety, alertness, and an appreciation of each other's tasks, during each shift, the two interior guards may alternate duties so that one guard does not have to make all of the watchclock tours or all of the random tours.

EMERGENCY CALLS

1. The touring guard winds all watchclock stations.
2. The walking guard travels the hospital at random, concentrating on critical areas and answering problem calls and emergency calls.
3. If it is necessary to call the police, it shall always be done through the hospital telephone operator.
4. All outside telephone calls should be made through the operator.

STRANGERS

A. Unknown
   1. All people in unusual places whom the guard does not recognize are to be challenged as to identification and reason for presence in that particular location.
   2. Unauthorized solicitors are to be ushered off hospital property.
   3. Use courtesy, intelligence, and tact.

B. Dangerous
   1. An armed intruder is the business of the police.
   2. Always use sound judgment when confronting any intruder.
   3. If an intruder appears to be armed, do not hesitate to call the police as quickly as possible through the telephone operator, but always keep the intruder in sight; use walkie-talkies.
   4. Guards are not to carry loaded firearms within the hospital building. (See also Memorandum Re: Armed Guards.)

VACATING POSTS

1. Guards are not to leave the hospital to open doors at interns' residence or doctors' building, but they are to respond to emergency call from either location.
2. Guards are not to vacate their posts until properly relieved.

ENDING SHIFTS

1. During the regular Monday through Friday workweek, the keys, walkie-talkie, and log sheets are to be turned in to the maintenance foreman at 8:00 a.m.

2. On weekends and holidays, the keys, walkie-talkie, and log sheets are turned over to the guards of the next shift.
3. All guards should punch out on the time clock with the same cards they punched in on—*after* their relief guards have punched in.

MISCELLANEOUS QUESTIONS

1. If ever there is a question of what to do, consult by telephone with the following:
   a. night mechanic (Page through the operator.)
   b. assistant administrative engineer
   c. administrative engineer
   d. director of engineering services
2. If there is a question about a patient or a visitor to a patient, consult with the following:
   a. nursing supervisor (Page through the operator.)
   b. administrator on call (by telephone)

SPECIAL INSTRUCTIONS

ALARMS

There are numerous alarms, bells and signal lights throughout the hospital. If one is activated, do not shut it off, but contact immediately the mechanics on duty.

EKG ROOM

The electrocardiograph room is not to be unlocked for anyone except the nursing supervisor or the administrator on call.

LAUNDRY

The guard will receive a call from either the nursing supervisor or a unit manager. The guard should unlock the laundry, for that person, record the items in the log as they are taken, and lock the door when all is complete.

LOADING PLATFORM DOOR (Receiving Dock)

Receiving department personnel are to lock their door at 5:00 p.m. every weekday. Security is to check this door hourly to make sure that it is secure.

If ever a delivery arrives when the door is locked, the telephone operator may direct security to unlock the door and to stand by until the delivery is complete. The guard should log such an occasion and secure the door when the delivery has been made.

MAILROOM

The mailroom should not be opened without approval of the information and mail supervisor, who should be contacted through the operator or the administrator on call. Note such action in the log.

MAINTENANCE STOCKROOM (Emergency Supplies)

Any individual who needs material from the maintenance stockroom during other than normal working hours must obtain permission from the shop foreman, assistant administrative engineer, or the administrative engineer, by telephone with the telephone operator and the security guard listening in. If such permission is granted, the guard will obtain the key to the stockroom from the telephone operator and will sign the key log sheet, indicating the time the key was taken.

The guard and the requesting individual will then proceed to the stockroom. Items removed must be listed on a repair request form and verified by the security guard. The key will then be returned to the telephone operator. Return of the key and time returned will be noted on the key log sheet. The security guard will enter this occurrence on the log sheet.

RUBBISH PACKER

The outside receiving door is to remain locked from 5:30 p.m. until 7:00 a.m. every weekday and all night and day on weekends. Housekeeping and dietary personnel making trash deposits after hours will use keys issued by maintenance. Their schedule usually runs until 11:00 p.m.

STOREROOM (Emergency Supplies)

The guard will be paged by the administrator on call and, with the telephone operator listening, be requested to accompany the person in need of emergency supplies into the storeroom. The guard will meet the person at the door to the telephone switchboard. They will knock to obtain the key, and the person seeking supplies will sign for the key with the guard standing by. The two of them will then go to the storeroom.

Items removed from the storeroom must be listed on a green emergency request form (found on the storekeeper's desk) by the person obtaining the items. The guard also must sign the green form. The key should be returned to the switchboard with the guard standing by as the person signs the logbook again. The guard should note in the log the time and the person accompanied to the storeroom.

SWITCHBOARD

If you must talk with the telephone operator, knock or call by telephone. Do not use your key.

FIRE

IF YOU DISCOVER ANY FIRE, ANY SIZE:

1. Never say "Fire!" Say "Drill" instead.
2. Pull the alarm box nearest the fire.
3. Dial operator and give exact location of drill including building and floor. Hold on until operator verifies location.
4. Close all doors and windows in the area including corridor doors.
5. Use proper fire extinguishers.

IF SOMEONE ELSE DISCOVERS A FIRE:

1. You will know that a drill is taking place when the alarm rings.
2. Make sure you know the exact location by reading the card next to fire alarm box.
3. If the fire is in the nurses' hall, the guard on duty there will remain and aid evacuating residents. If the fire is in the north or south building, the guard should call and inform the elevator operator (in the north or south building) of the fire drill and its location. The elevator operator should be instructed to land the elevator on the first floor, hold the elevator until firefighters arrive, and take them to the drill location.
4. If there is no guard on duty in the nurses' hall, both interior guards should meet at the scene of the drill and immediately decide which exterior door is the most direct entrance for firefighters. If the fire is in the north or south building, one guard should call and inform the elevator operator concerned of the fire drill and its location. The elevator operator should be instructed to land the elevator on the first floor, hold the elevator until firefighters arrive, and take them to the drill location. This guard should then go quickly to the proper outside door, unlock it if necessary, and direct the firefighters to the waiting elevator.
5. The main entrance guard shall ascertain location of the drill, and stand by outside to clear any traffic obstructing the passage of incoming fire apparatus. The guard should also direct fire apparatus through the driveway that is most appropriate for fast access to the drill location.

The "All Clear" signal consists of four short rings with a long pause between each ring.

DISASTER

By hospital definition, a "disaster" is a situation in which the number of patients arriving is judged to be in excess of the normal load. Notification of a disaster situation will come from the telephone operator or by "0" appearing on the doctors' call register with a gong. The primary duty of the security force during a disaster is to direct incoming patients into the main building lobby rather than the emergency ward. Further instructions will come from the senior person in the maintenance department.

WALKING PATROLS

Guards are to walk (roam) the complete hospital—all buildings—with the exception of the inpatient areas, which are not to be entered on any tour, except when specific aid is requested or in case of fire. Nurses' residence areas in nurses' hall are not to be entered during the 4:30 p.m. and 7:30 p.m. tours, unless specific aid is requested or in case of fire.

MONDAY–FRIDAY
Tour #1
(4:00 p.m./1600 Hours)

4:00 p.m. (Monday-Friday): One guard escorts cashier from the OPD lobby to cashier's office in main lobby.

One guard begins locking exterior doors in accordance with Schedule 1 (See page 94.) Interior doors are to be locked according to Schedule 2 (See page 95.)

Do not wind watch stations on this tour. Do make yourself available to people along your routes who may have special instructions for you and note them in your log.

Do not lock offices, laboratories, etc., that are left open since hospital personnel may still be working (this tour only).

Do not enter the operating suite.

The other interior guard should be roaming the hospital, ready to answer any problem calls promptly.

Tour #2
(7:30 p.m./1930 Hours)

One guard winds all watch stations and checks all doors. If no one is working in an area, the lights should be turned off and the doors locked.

The other interior guard should be roaming the hospital, ready to answer any problem calls promptly.

Tour #3

(10:00 p.m./2200 Hours)

One guard winds all watch stations, checks all doors and locks and logs any doors found unlocked. The other interior guard should be roaming the hospital, ready to answer any problem calls promptly.

(10:45 p.m./2245 Hours)

One guard should open all basement and first-floor laboratories and offices in the nurses' hall one at a time to check window locks. If any windows are found open or unlocked, they should be closed, locked, and logged. Then the door should be locked as the guard leaves. This should be completed by 11:30 p.m. (2330 Hours), when the housemother goes off duty.

(11:30 p.m./2330 Hours)

One guard should report to the front entrance of the nurses' hall to relieve the housemother. This guard is responsible for allowing only residents of the nurses' hall to enter the building and should ask any unfamiliar person for identification. This post shall be manned until 8:00 a.m. (0800 Hours).

Tour #4

(12:30 a.m./0030 Hours)

One guard begins winding all watch stations. All doors should be checked. If any are found open, they should be locked and the room number logged. The other interior guard should be stationed at the nurses' hall entrance.

Tour #5

(2:30 a.m./0230 Hours)

One guard begins winding all watch stations, locking all open doors, and logging them. The other interior guard should be stationed at the nurses' hall entrance.

Tour #6

(5:00 a.m./0500 Hours)

One guard winds all watch stations, checking all doors, locking and logging the doors found open. Exterior doors should be unlocked by one guard in accordance with Schedule #3 on page 93. Interior doors should be unlocked by one guard in accordance with Schedule #4 on page 93. The other guard should be stationed at the nurses' hall entrance.

SATURDAYS, SUNDAYS, AND HOLIDAYS
Tour #7
(8:30 a.m./0830 Hours)

One guard winds all watch stations, checking all doors, and locking and logging any doors found open. The other interior guard should be roaming the hospital, ready to answer any problem calls promptly.

Tour #8
(10:30 a.m./1030 Hours)

One guard winds all watch stations, checking all doors, locking and logging any doors found open. The other interior guard should be roaming the hospital, ready to answer any problem calls promptly.

Tour #9
(12:30 p.m./1230 Hours)

One guard winds all watch stations, checks all doors, and locks and logs any doors found open. The other interior guard should be roaming the hospital, ready to answer any problem calls promptly.

Tour #10
(2:30 a.m./1430 Hours)

One guard winds all watch stations, checks all doors, and locks and logs any doors found open. The other interior guard should be roaming the hospital, ready to answer any problem call promptly.

EXTERIOR DOOR LOCKING SCHEDULE
LOCK-UP/SCHEDULE #1

Door Locations	Mon.-Fri.	Saturday	Sunday	Holidays
1. Side Entrance	1630	1300	All Day	All Day
2. North Building Rear	1700	—	Locked All Day	—
3. Receiving Dock		See Special Instructions Page 00		
4. Rear of Building "A"	1700	—	Locked All Day	—
5. Refrigeration Plant Ext. Door	1700	—	Locked All Day	—

6. Rubbish Packer		See Special Instructions Page 00		
7. South Building Rear Exit	1800	—	Locked All Day	—
8. Memorial Auditorium	1800	—	Check Schedule	—
9. Research Front Exit	1800	—	Locked All Day	—
10. Research Rear Exit	1800	—	Locked All Day	—
11. Nurses' Hall Rear Exit South	1800	—	Locked All Day	—
12. Nurses' Hall Rear Exit North	1830	—	Locked All Day	—
13. South Building Employees' Exit	1830	1830	1830	1830
14. Employees' Auditorium Exit	1830	—	Locked All Day	—
15. Tunnel to Nurses' Hall	2200	2200	2200	2200

INTERIOR DOOR LOCKING SCHEDULE
LOCK-UP/SCHEDULE #2

Door Location	Mon.-Fri.	Saturday	Sunday	Holidays
1. CB-391 Radiation Therapy	1800	—	Locked All Day	—
2. C4701 Stair	1800	—	Locked All Day	—
3. C3701 Stair	1800	—	Locked All Day	—
4. C2701 Stair	1800	—	Locked All Day	—
5. Second Floor to Building C	1800	—	Locked All Day	—
6. C184A Stair	1800	—	Locked All Day	—
7. Rear of Employees'	1800	—	Locked All Day	—
8. 4th Floor East Wing to Building C	1800	—	Locked All Day	—
9. C473B Stair	1800	—	Locked All Day	—
10. C372B Stair	1800	—	Locked All Day	—
11. C373B to Building C	1800	—	Locked All Day	—
12. C273B Stair	1800	—	Locked All Day	—
13. C180B Stair	1800	—	Locked All Day	—

EXTERIOR DOOR UNLOCKING SCHEDULE
UNLOCK/SCHEDULE #3

Door Location	Mon.-Fri.	Saturday	Sunday	Holidays
1. South Building Employees' Entrance	0500	0500	0500	0500
2. North Building Front	0600	—	Locked All Day	—
3. Receiving Dock		See Special Instructions Page 00		
4. Tunnel Nurses' Hall	0600	0600	0600	0600
5. Nurses' Hall Rear North	0600	0600	0600	0600
6. Nurses' Hall Rear South	0700	—	Locked All Day	—
7. Research Front	0700	—	Locked All Day	—
8. Research Rear	0700	—	Locked All Day	—
9. Main Entrance	0700	0730	Lock	Lock
10. North Building Rear	0700	—	Locked All Day	—
11. Rubbish Packer		See Special Instructions Page 00		
12. Building C Rear	0700	—	Locked All Day	—
13. Memorial Auditorium	0700	—	Check Schedule	—
14. South Building Rear	0730	—	Locked All Day	—

INTERIOR DOOR UNLOCKING SCHEDULE
UNLOCK/SCHEDULE #4

Door Location	Mon.-Fri.	Saturday	Sunday	Holidays
1. C4701 Stair	0700	—	Locked All Day	—
2. C3701 Stair	0700	—	Locked All Day	—
3. C2701 Stair	0700	—	Locked All Day	—
4. Second Floor to Building L	0700	—	Locked All Day	—
5. C184A	0700	—	Locked All Day	—
6. Rear of Memorial	0700	—	Locked All Day	—
7. 4th Floor East Wing to Building C	0700	—	Locked All Day	—
8. C473B Stair	0700	—	Locked All Day	—
9. C372B Stair	0700	—	Locked All Day	—
10. C373B to Building C	0700	—	Locked All Day	—
11. C273B Stair	0700	—	Locked All Day	—
12. C180B Stair	0700	—	Locked All Day	—
13. CB-391 Radiation Therapy	0730	—	Locked All Day	—

KEYS ON #1 & #2 GUARD RINGS

1. L & R Master
2. Main Master
3. Research Master
4. OPD Master
5. South & Service Master
6. North Master
7. Memorial Master
8. Emergency Exit Locks
9. Emergency Exit Locks, Nurses' Hall
10. 3 Subbasements
11. Main Entrance
12. Memorial Main Entrance
13. Mortise Square Key
14. Nurses' Hall Basement
15. Nurses' Hall Basement
16. Nurses' Hall 2nd Floor Master

Housemother's keys (transferred to the nurses' hall guard when housemother goes off duty):

1. Personnel Offices
2. Old Annex 2nd Floor
3. Old Annex 3rd Floor
4. Old Annex 4th Floor
5. "New Annex" Master
6. Closet Master "New Annex"
7. Nurses' Hall Basement
8. Nurses' Hall 2nd Floor Master

WATCHMAN'S CLOCK STATIONS

Research Building		*OPD*	
Penthouse	151	Penthouse	251
4th Floor	141	3rd Floor	231
3rd Floor	131	2nd Floor	221
2nd Floor	121	1st Floor	211
1st Floor	111	Basement	201
Subbasement	101	Basement	202

Nurses' Hall

4th Floor	341
4th Floor	342
3rd Floor	331
3rd Floor	332
2nd Floor	321
2nd Floor	322
1st Floor	311
1st Floor	312
Basement	301
Basement	302
Basement	303

Main Building

Penthouse	451
4th Floor	441
3rd Floor	431
3rd Floor	432
2nd Floor	421
2nd Floor	422
1st Floor	411
1st Floor	412
1st Floor	413
Basement	401
Basement	402

North and East Bldgs.

4th Floor	541
3rd Floor	531
3rd Floor	532
2nd Floor	521
2nd Floor	522
1st Floor	511
1st Floor	512
Basement	501
Basement	502
Basement	503
Subbasement	504

South and Service Bldgs.

3rd Floor	631
2nd Floor	621
2nd Floor	622
1st Floor	611
Basement	601
Basement	602
Subbasement	603
Subbasement	604

L and R Buildings

4th Floor	741
4th Floor	742
4th Floor	743
3rd Floor	731
3rd Floor	732
3rd Floor	733
2nd Floor	721
2nd Floor	722
2nd Floor	723
1st Floor	711
1st Floor	712
1st Floor	713
Basement	701
Basement	702
Subbasement	703
Subbasement	704
Subbasement	705

Refrigeration Plant

Basement	801
Subbasement	802

Service Building

Penthouse	641
Penthouse	642

USE THESE NUMBERS WHEN REFERRING TO A
STATION LOCATION

STATIC POSTS

MAIN ENTRANCE POST

At 9:00 p.m. (2100 Hours), when posted at the main entrance of the hospital, the guard should check in with the operator and fill out the heading of the log report. This post is to be manned until 8:00 a.m. (0800 Hours). Surveillance of the inner parking area is the main duty of this post, although the guard is also responsible for all hospital grounds at the Main Street location. The guard is also to escort personnel leaving the hospital through the main entrance to their cars or to Main Street if they ask for assistance.

The guard at the main entrance is the only guard on duty outside of the hospital and shall focus attention on the outdoor areas of the hospital. The other two guards should survey the hospital's interior. Only in emergencies should either of the two interior guards accompany the main entrance guard out of doors.

If an armed intruder should appear on the hospital grounds, the guard should immediately notify the police through the telephone operator and use proper judgement in confronting such an intruder.

All unusual situations must be noted by the guard in the log which is to be given to the maintenance shop foreman each weekday morning at 8:00 a.m. (0800 Hours). On weekend and holiday mornings, the log is turned over to the relief.

During a fire drill, it shall be the responsibility of the main entrance guard to direct firefighters to the scene of the fire and to direct any other traffic out of the way of incoming fire apparatus. This responsibility should be shared with one of the other two guards.

During the time of a disaster, the main entrance guard will direct traffic at the main entrance and keep it clear for ambulances coming into the front of the emergency room.

NURSES' QUARTERS GUARD

At 10:45 p.m. (2245 Hours)—One guard should open all basement and first-floor laboratories and offices (except dark room in KB-10) in the nurses' hall, one at a time, to check window locks. If any windows are found open or unlocked, they should be closed, locked and logged. Then the door should be locked as the guard leaves. This should be completed by 11:30 p.m. (2330 Hours).

At 11:30 p.m. (2330 Hours)—One guard reports to the front entrance of the nurses' hall (Personnel's Reception Office) to relieve the housemother. This guard, or the alternate at the post, is responsible for allowing only residents of the nurses' hall to enter the building and challenging any un-familiar person.

At 12:00 p.m. (2400 Hours) an exchange of guard is effected as the 1600-to 2400-hour guard is relieved of the nurses' hall post by the 0100-0800-hour guard, who carries the same responsibilities. This post is not to be vacated until a relief arrives. This post shall be manned until 0800 Hours. (See page 91 concerning fire drill procedures.)

TIME CONVERSION TABLE

1:00 a.m.	0100 Hours	1:00 p.m.	1300 Hours
2:00 a.m.	0200 Hours	2:00 p.m.	1400 Hours
3:00 a.m.	0300 Hours	3:00 p.m.	1500 Hours
4:00 a.m.	0400 Hours	4:00 p.m.	1600 Hours
5:00 a.m.	0500 Hours	5:00 p.m.	1700 Hours
6:00 a.m.	0600 Hours	6:00 p.m.	1800 Hours
7:00 a.m.	0700 Hours	7:00 p.m.	1900 Hours
8:00 a.m.	0800 Hours	8:00 p.m.	2000 Hours
9:00 a.m.	0900 Hours	9:00 p.m.	2100 Hours
10:00 a.m.	1000 Hours	10:00 p.m.	2200 Hours
11:00 a.m.	1100 Hours	11:00 p.m.	2300 Hours
12:00 Noon	1200 Hours	12:00 Midnight	2400 Hours

1:30 a.m.	0130 Hours	12:59 a.m.	0059 Hours
2:45 a.m.	0245 Hours	11:52 p.m.	2352 Hours
3:43 p.m.	1543 Hours	10:03 a.m.	1003 Hours
12:45 a.m.	0045 Hours	10:03 p.m.	2203 Hours

MEMORANDUM

To: Security Guards   Date: August 2

From: Director of Security

Re: Armed Guard

1. Any Guard or Supervisor that is armed and at Memorial Hospital, whether to stand guard or on inspections, will not carry a loaded weapon in the interior of the Hospital when called into any patient area or to an emergency.

2. The weapon that is carried by the Guard patrolling the outside grounds is the only weapon to be carried anywhere on Hospital property.

3. If at any time a problem arises at any other point inside the Hospital, no person shall draw a weapon for any reason. By doing so, it is cause for immediate suspension and possible loss of job.

4. Any time a guard is called into the Hospital:
   a. Weapon shall be unloaded before entering.
   b. Weapon shall be put into pants pocket.
   c. Weapon will not be taken out until emergency is over and guard is back at post outside Hospital.
   d. Weapon is not to be left anywhere or given to anyone to hold.

MEMORANDUM

To: Security Guards   Date: August 6

From: Administrative Engineer

Re: Time Cards

As of this notice, security guards will begin using the maintenance department's time clock.

Six time cards have been made up:

Two	4:00 p.m. to 12:00 midnight shift
Two	12:00 Midnight to 8:00 a.m. shift
Two	8:00 a.m. to 4:00 p.m. shift

The latter pair of cards will be used only on Saturdays, Sundays, and holidays as we have no day shift of guards during the regular workweek.

The cards belong to the shift, not to each individual guard. Therefore, each guard is to do the following:

1. Punch in and out, using one or the other of the pair of cards for your shift.
2. SIGN YOUR NAME next to the day and time which the time clock prints on the card.

If there are any questions, see me.

MEMORANDUM

To: Security Guards   August 31

From: Assistant Administrative Engineer

Re: 200 Parkway — Policy regarding an incident

200 Parkway is the six-story residence for dietary aides and other female employees which is located north of the hospital on the corner of the Parkway and Main Street.

It has been previously stressed that guards are not to leave the hospital grounds — particularly to open doors for someone who lost her key. The introduction of the two-way radio and recent incidents at and around 200 Parkway dictate the following modification to the policy:

1. Guards will be issued a key to the front door of 200 Parkway.
2. Whenever an incident is reported at 200 Parkway, the police will be called at once through the telephone operator.
3. The security guard who is making walking rounds, while in radio contact with the other guards, should proceed to the scene and act as the hospital representative.
4. The security guard so acting shall record all pertinent details in the log, which will be the official record of the event.
5. If there is a security guard already on call at 200 Parkway and further need arises at the Hospital, the guard will immediately return to the hospital.
6. Contact should be maintained via the two-way radio at all times.

MEMORANDUM

To: Security Guards   Date: August 17

From: Administrative Engineer

Re: Lights and Doors

Please put all regular lights in all basement service and research building corridors out at 5:00 p.m. as you make your first round, thus leaving on only the emergency lights. Also, reduce light level in other corridors at 9:00 p.m. and after 12:00 midnight as housekeeper tends to leave lights on after clean-up.

During the other rounds please try the doors to all laboratories and offices to be sure that they are locked. If the door is found open after your first round, please note this in your log book.

MEMORANDUM

To: All Maintenance Personnel   Date: March 13
       All Security Personnel

From: Administrative Engineer

       Re: ALARM SYSTEM

The importance of alarms cannot be overemphasized. If *any* alarm signal (light, bell, buzzer, etc.) is encountered, *do not* ignore it. They all mean something.

The security personnel should notify the hospital mechanic on duty who, in turn, should take the necessary action to correct the trouble indicated.

If there is any doubt as to what action to take, call for advice or assistance through the operator.

If a service company is called and it fails to respond within a reasonable time, call again. If there is an unreasonable delay or no response, call for assistance as noted in the above paragraph.
It must be stated again:

DO NOT IGNORE ALARMS!

SPECIAL FIRE REGULATIONS
FOR SECURITY GUARDS

(11:30 p.m. — 8:00 a.m.)

When the fire alarm sounds or when informed of a fire by the telephone operator, determine exact location.

1. If the drill is in the nurses' hall, the nurses' hall guard shall aid residents in evacuation from the building. The other guard shall determine the exact location of the drill and direct incoming fire department personnel to the hospital entrance which is the most direct for access to the drill location.

2. If the drill is in the north or south buildings, the nurses' hall guard shall remain at the post and call the elevator operator concerned (North Building 577 and South Building 495), inform the operator of the fire drill and its location, and instruct the operator to land the elevator at the first floor to wait for the firefighters and transport them to the drill location.

Approved: _____

Section
-8E-

Distribution:
  Safety & Fire Manual

Effective: _____

Replaces: _____

SPECIAL FIRE INSTRUCTIONS FOR THE MAIN ENTRANCE

INFORMATION DESK — 7:00 a.m.-9:00 p.m.

Upon being notified of a fire by the telephone operator or by hearing the fire alarm signals, count signals and determine location on code signal card.

1. Stand by outside to notify the parking lot attendant to clear the traffic circle, and direct the fire department personnel to the exact location of the fire. Be sure to use the bull horn so that you may be heard clearly.
2. Have all visitors wait in the main lobby, until the "All Clear" has been sounded.

GUARD AT MAIN ENTRANCE — 9:00 p.m.-7:00 a.m.

Upon being notified of the location of a fire by the telephone operator or by hearing the fire alarm signals, count signals and determine location on code signal card.

1. Stand by outside and clear the traffic circle for incoming fire apparatus and direct the fire department personnel through the most appropriate driveway for quickly reaching the location of the drill. Use the bull horn (located at the information desk) so that you may be heard clearly.
2. All visitors are to be directed to wait in the main lobby, until the "All Clear" has been sounded.

Approved: _____

Section
-8C-

Distribution:

Effective: _____

Safety & Fire Manual

Replaces: _____

PATROLS

In addition to manning stationary posts, security officers will also be responsible for patrolling various areas on a routine basis to check for intruders and to ensure the proper maintenance of fire prevention and general safety standards. Patrol responsibilities can include anything from turning light switches on and off to whatever job management feels is necessary and the director of security approves. Usually, security officers assigned to patrol duty have basic responsibilities for maintaining fire and safety inspections and reporting on any violations of policies or procedures that their patrols uncover.

The reports of the patrol officers, although routinely dull, can produce very important information and can alert the security section to potential trouble. The reports should be submitted on a per-officer-shift basis and should be of the narrative, rather than the format, type (see Chapter 7). They should provide an hourly account of areas covered and situations revealed during the scheduled rounds. There are a few "foolproof" systems on the market to authenticate the rounds made by the patrol officer. However, only when coupled with an hourly narrative report to be submitted by each security officer as each shift expires, will any of these systems ensure proper coverage.

Patrol officers who begin to decide on their own when and how often they are going to perform specific patrols should be watched carefully. Such self-made decisions usually conflict with instructions.

All officers assigned to patrol must be physically and mentally equipped to perform the patrol efficiently; their conditions must be checked periodically. For example, an older officer incapable of direct physical contact should not patrol a section of the facility in which it might be necessary physically to subdue patients. The same officer could, however, be used very effectively in a patrol involving only maintenance checks on empty portions of the building.

Facility management must take steps to assure that the assigned patrol has been carried out as directed. This can be accomplished in many ways; one of the most efficient is placing alarm boxes in strategic areas of the building or patrol area. The patrolling officer then, in the course of the round, takes the key found at each strategic area and, by inserting it in the alarm box clock, records the time that the specific area was covered. Similarly, if equipment such as fire extinguishers needs to be checked periodically, the security officer should be directed to sign and date the card attached to the equipment. These cards should be affixed with sealing wax and stamped. Too many times they are removed at the start of a shift and replaced at the end of the shift. Supervisory checks are necessary to ensure compliance with these authenticating procedures.

One of the most important elements of supervising patrol officers is the monitoring of their attitudes. A patrol officer must never develop a hostile, Gestapo-like attitude toward suspected intruders apprehended during patrol rounds. Experience has proven that there is no need for this type of tactic, and suits can be brought against the facility if a suspected intruder is treated badly. Every situation must be handled in a rational manner. The very first indication of a guard's belligerent attitude should be grounds for a corrective interview. The officer should be informed that if the incorrect attitude is not corrected within a specific length of time, dismissal will result. Any officer whose attitude does not improve should be advised that such behavior can no longer be tolerated, and dismissed. In this same vein, the security officer who mechanically fulfills the assigned rounds but spends most of the time socializing with other personnel is a similar hazard to the force and should be removed as soon as possible.

Under no circumstances should a person who has been employed by security be allowed to go to work in another section of the hospital. I do not feel that this rule should apply to the security officers who perform the security responsibilities well and who have proven that they are worthy of remaining on the payroll of the facility. I speak here primarily of the security officers who do not perform their duties as they should. There might be future problems if they are reassigned to other jobs in the facility, especially since they would have the knowledge of the entire workings of the security department.

A record must be maintained on everything that the security officer does in the route of the patrol tour. The record must be a coordinated effort whereby any item requiring attention by anybody other than security supervision be maintained and a copy forwarded to the appropriate department. For example, the patrol supervisor should prepare a work order asking that the maintenance department fix any maintenance problem discovered by the patrol. Items not in the realm of the maintenance supervisor's responsibility should be reported to the administrator via a similar type of form. Items of a serious nature involving top management should be sent directly to the director of security, who can notify the appropriate facility official. See Chapter 7 for detailed information on proper security report form and situations requiring security reports.

Appendix A

Bomb Threats and Search Techniques*

*Prepared by the U.S. Department of the Treasury, Bureau of Alcohol, Tobacco and Firearms, Washington, D.C. 20226. Reprinted with permission.

Foreword

Bombing and the threat of bombing have created a need for practical knowledge to cope with the increasingly violent activities of people who represent segments of unrest in our society. Repeated criminal acts which use or threaten to use explosives against educational institutions, industry, law enforcement and the general public, place a most urgent responsibility on law enforcement agencies. However, the protection of life and property is a responsibility that cannot be delegated to law enforcement alone. Every citizen must be prepared to accept responsibility if we are to enjoy a safe place in which to live and work.

Information for the preparation of this document was obtained from a wide range of official and private sources, including the actual experience of Alcohol, Tobacco and Firearms Special Agents. The ideas and methods suggested reflect the most current information available to help you.

One suggestion in this document should be emphasized; it is preparedness. When one is equipped with an organized plan, most bomb threat problems can be resolved with minimal personal injury and property damage.

By making this "Bomb Threats and Search Techniques" available to selected persons, we in ATF are attempting to help you help yourself in dealing with bomb threats and the use of explosives for illegal purposes.

Rex D. Davis

REX D. DAVIS, DIRECTOR
BUREAU OF ALCOHOL, TOBACCO AND FIREARMS

Purpose of Calls

The only two reasonable explanations for a call reporting that a bomb is to go off in a particular installation are:

1

The caller has definite knowledge or believes that an explosive or incendiary has been or will be placed and he wants to minimize personal injury or property damage. The caller may be the person who placed the device or someone else who has become aware of such information.

2

The caller wants to create an atmosphere of anxiety and panic which will, in turn, possibly result in a disruption of the normal activities at the installation where the device is purportedly located.

When a bomb threat call has been received, there will be a reaction to it. If the call is directed to an installation where a vacuum of leadership exists or where there has been no organized advance planning to handle such threats, the call will result in panic.

Panic

Panic is one of the most contagious of all human emotions. Panic is defined as a "sudden, excessive, unreasoning, infectious terror." Panic is caused by fear—fear of the known or the unknown. Panic can also be defined in the context of a bomb threat call as the ultimate achievement of the caller.

Once a state of panic has been reached, the potential for personal injury and property damage is dramatically increased. Emergency and essential facilities can be shut down or abandoned and the community denied their use at a critical time.

Leaving facilities unattended can lead to destruction of the facility and the surrounding area. Large chemical manufacturing plants, power plants, unattended boilers, and other such facilities require the attention of operating personnel.

Other effects of not being prepared or not having an organized plan to handle bomb threat calls can result in a lack of confidence in the leadership. This will be reflected in lower productivity or reluctance to continue employment at a location that is being subjected to bomb threat calls.

Preparation

Lines of organization and plans must be made in advance to handle bomb threats. Clear-cut levels of authority must be established. It is important that each person handle his assignment without delay and without any signs of fear.

Only by using an established organization and procedures can you handle these problems with the least risk. This will instill confidence and eliminate panic.

In planning, you should designate a control center or command post. This control center should be located in the switchboard room or other focal point of telephone or radio communications. The management personnel assigned to operate the control center should have decision-making authority on the action to be taken during the threat. Reports on the progress of the search and evacuation should be made to the control center. Only those with assigned duties should be permitted in the control center. Make some provision for alternates in the event someone is absent when the threat is received.

Evacuation

The most serious of all decisions to be made by management in the event of a bomb threat is evacuation or non-evacuation of the building.

The decision to evacuate or not to evacuate may be made during the planning phase. Management may pronounce a carte blanche policy that in the event of a bomb threat, evacuation will be effected immediately. This decision circumvents the calculated risk and gives prime consideration for the safety of personnel in the building. This can result in production down-time, and can be costly, if the threat is a hoax. The alternative is for management to make the decision on the spot at the time of the threat. There is no magic formula which can produce the proper decision.

In the past, the vast majority of bomb threats turned out to be hoaxes. However, today more of the threats are materializing. Thus, management's first consideration must be for the safety of people. It is practically impossible to determine immediately whether a bomb threat is real.

Investigations have revealed that the targets for "terrorist bombings" are not selected at random. The modus operandi for selecting the target(s) and planting the explosive appears to follow this pattern. The target is selected because of political or personal gain to the terrorist. It is then kept under surveillance to determine the entrances and exits most used, and when. This is done to determine the hours when very few people are in the building. The idea is that the intent is not to injure or kill people, but to destroy the building. Reconnaissance of the building is made to locate an area where a bomb can be concealed, do the most damage, and where the "bomber" is least likely to be observed.

A test, or dry run, of the plan is often made. After the "dry run" and at a predetermined time, the building is infiltrated by the "bomber(s)" to deliver the explosives or incendiary device. The device may be fully or partially pre-set prior to planting. If it is fully set and charged, it is a simple matter for one or two of the group to plant the device in a pre-selected concealed area. This can be accomplished in a minimum of time. If the device is not fully set and charged, one member may act as a lookout while others arm and place the device. Most devices used for the destruction of property are usually of the time-delay type. These devices can be

set for detonation to allow sufficient time for the "bomber(s)" to be a considerable distance away before the bomb-threat call is made and the device is detonated.

The terrorists have developed their plan of attack and the following procedures are suggested to business and industry for coping with bomb threats.

How to Prepare

1
Contact the police, fire department or other local governmental agencies to determine whether any has a bomb disposal unit. Under what conditions is the bomb disposal unit available? What is the telephone number? How can you obtain the services of the bomb disposal unit in the event of a bomb threat? Will the bomb disposal unit assist in the physical search of the building or will they only disarm or remove explosives?

2
Establish strict procedures for control and inspection of packages and material entering critical areas.

3
Develop a positive means of identifying and controlling personnel who are authorized access to critical areas.

4
Arrange, if possible, to have police and/or fire representatives with members of your staff inspect the building for areas where explosives are likely to be concealed. This may be accomplished by reviewing the floor plan of the building.

5
During the inspection of the building, you should give particular attention to elevator shafts, all ceiling areas, rest rooms, access doors, and crawl space in rest rooms and areas used as access to plumbing fixtures, electrical fixtures, utility and other closet areas, space under stairwells, boiler (furnace) rooms, flammable storage areas, main switches and valves, e.g., electric, gas, and fuel, indoor trash receptacles, record storage

areas, mail rooms, ceiling lights with easily removable panels, and fire hose racks. While this list is not complete, it can give you an idea where a time-delayed explosive or an incendiary device may be concealed.

6

All security and maintenance personnel should be alert to suspicious looking or unfamiliar persons or objects.

7

You should instruct security and maintenance personnel to make periodic checks of all rest rooms, stairwells, under stairwells, and other areas of the building to assure that unauthorized personnel are not hiding or reconnoitering or surveilling the area.

8

You should assure adequate protection for classified documents, proprietary information and other records essential to the operation of your business. A well-planted, properly charged device could, upon detonation, destroy those records needed in day-to-day operations. Computers have also been singled out as targets by bombers.

9

Instruct all personnel, especially those at the telephone switchboard, in what to do if a bomb threat call is received.

As a minimum, every telephone operator or receptionist should be trained to respond calmly to a bomb threat call. To assist these individuals, a bomb threat call checklist of the type illustrated at the back of this pamphlet should be kept nearby. In addition, it is always desirable that more than one person listen in on the call. To do this, have a covert signalling system, perhaps a coded buzzer signal to a second reception point. A calm response to the bomb threat could result in getting additional information. This is especially true if the caller wishes to avoid injuries or deaths. If told that the building is occupied or cannot be evacuated in time, the bomber may be willing to give more specific information on the bomb's location.

10

Organize and train an evacuation unit consisting of key management personnel. The organization and training of this unit should be coordinated with other tenants of the building.

a The evacuation unit should be trained on how to evacuate the building during a bomb threat. You should consider priority of evacuation, i.e., evacuation by floor level. Evacuate the floor levels above the danger area in order to remove those persons from danger as quickly as possible. Training in this type of evacuation should be available from police, fire or other units within the community.

b You may also train the evacuation unit in search techniques, or you may prefer a separate search unit. Volunteer personnel should be solicited for this function. Assignment of search wardens, team leaders, etc. can be employed. To be proficient in searching the building, search personnel must be thoroughly familiar with all hallways, restrooms, false ceiling areas and every location in the building where an explosive or incendiary device may be concealed. When the police or firemen arrive at the building, if they have not previously reconnoitered the building, the contents and the floor plan will be strange to them. Thus, it is extremely important that the evacuation or search unit be thoroughly trained and familiar with the floor plan of the building and immediate outside areas. When the room or particular facility is searched it should be marked or the room sealed with a piece of tape and reported to the group supervisor.

c The evacuation or search unit should be trained only in evacuation and search techniques and not in the techniques of neutralizing, removing or otherwise having contact with the device. If a device is located it should not be disturbed but a string or paper tape may be run from the device location to a safe distance and used later as a guide to the device.

When A Bomb Threat Is Called In:

a **Keep the caller on the line as long as possible.** Ask him to repeat the message. Record every word spoken by the person.

b If the caller does not indicate the location of the bomb or the time of possible detonation, you should ask him for this information.

c Inform the caller that the building is occupied and the detonation of a bomb could result in death or serious injury to many innocent people.

d Pay particular attention to peculiar background noises such as, motors running, background music, and any other noise which may give a clue as to the location of the caller.

e Listen closely to the voice (male, female), voice quality (calm, excited), accents and speech impediments. Immediately after the caller hangs up, you should report to the person designated by management to receive such information. Since the law enforcement personnel will want to talk first-hand with the person who received the call, he should remain available until they appear.

f Report this information immediately to the police department, fire department, ATF, FBI, and other appropriate agencies. The sequence of notification should have been established during coordination in item 1 above.

Written Threats

Save all materials, including any envelope or container. Once the message is recognized as a bomb threat, further unnecessary handling should be avoided. Every possible effort must be made to retain evidence such as fingerprints, handwriting or typewriting, paper, and postal marks which are essential to tracing the threat and identifying the writer.

While written messages are usually associated with generalized threats and extortion attempts, a written warning of a specific device may occasionally be received. It should never be ignored. With the growing use of voice print identification techniques to identify and convict telephone callers, there may well be an increase in the use of written warnings and calls to third parties.

Bomb Search Techniques

a Do not touch a strange or suspicious object. Its location and description should be reported to the person designated to receive this information.

b The removal and disarming of a bomb or suspicious object must be left to the professionals in explosive ordnance disposal. Who these professionals are and how to contact them for assistance is something that you should include in any bomb threat plan.

c All requests for assistance should be directed to one or more of the Emergency Numbers listed on page three of this booklet. Be sure that the telephone numbers for these agencies are included in your plan.

d If the danger zone is located, the area should be blocked off or barricaded with a clear zone of three hundred feet until the object has been removed or disarmed.

e During the search of the building, a rapid two-way communication system is of utmost importance. Such a system can be readily established through existing telephones. CAUTION—the use of radios during the search can be dangerous. The radio transmission energy can cause premature detonation of an electric initiator (blasting cap).

f The signal for evacuating the building in the event of a bomb threat should not be the same as that for a fire. In the bomb threat, where possible, all doors and windows should be opened to permit the blast wave to escape in the event of an explosion. Also, evacuation routes will have to be determined if a bomb is found so as to lead people away from the bomb.

g If the building is evacuated, controls must be established immediately to prevent unauthorized access to the building. These controls may have to be provided by management. If proper coordination has been effected with the local police and other agencies, these may assist in establishing controls to prevent re-entry into the building until the danger has passed.

h Evacuate the persons to a safe distance away from the building to protect them against debris and other flying objects if there is an explosion. If the building is evacuated, all gas and fuel lines should be cut off at the main valve. All electrical equipment should be turned off prior to evacuation. The decision to cut off all electrical power at the main switch should be made by management with consideration given to lighting requirements for search teams.

i During the search, the medical personnel of the building should be alerted to stand by in case of an accident caused by an explosion of the device.

j Fire brigade personnel should be alerted to stand by to man fire extinguishers.

k Pre-emergency plans should include a temporary relocation in the event the bomb threat materializes and the building is determined to be unsafe.

Room Search

The following technique is based on use of a two-man searching team. There are many minor variations possible in searching a room. The following contains only the basic techniques.

First Team Action—listening

When the two-man search team enters the room to be searched, they should first move to various parts of the room and stand quietly, with their eyes shut and listen for a clock-work device. Frequently, a clock-work mechanism can be quickly detected without use of special equipment. Even if no clockwork mechanism is detected, the team is now aware of the background noise level within the room itself.

Background noise or transferred sound is always disturbing during a building search. In searching a building, if a ticking sound is heard but cannot be located, one might become unnerved. The ticking sound may come from an unbalanced air conditioner fan several floors away or from a dripping sink down the hall. Sound will transfer through air-conditioning ducts, along water pipes and through walls, etc. One of the worst types of buildings to work in is one that has steam or water heat. This type of building will constantly thump, crack, chatter and tick due to the movement of the steam or hot water through the pipes and the expansion and contraction of the pipes. Background noise may also be outside traffic sounds, rain, wind, etc.

Second Team Action—Division of Room and Selection of Search Height

The man in charge of the room searching team should look around the room and determine how the room is to be divided for searching and to what height the first searching sweep should extend. The first searching sweep will cover all items resting on the floor up to the selected height.

Dividing The Room. You should divide the room into two equal parts or as nearly equal as possible. This equal division should be based on the number and type of objects in the room to be searched, not the size of the room. An imaginary line is then drawn between two objects in the room, i.e., the edge of the window on the north wall to the floor lamp on the south wall.

Selection of First Searching Height. Look at the furniture or objects in the room and determine the average height of the majority of items resting on the floor. In an average room this height usually includes table or desk tops, chair backs, etc. The first searching height usually covers the items in the room up to hip height.

First Room Searching Sweep

After the room has been divided and a searching height has been selected, both men go to one end of the room division line and start from a back-to-back position. This is the starting point, and the same point will be used on each successive searching sweep. Each man now starts searching his way around the room, working toward the other man, checking all items resting on the floor around the wall area of the room. When the two men meet, they will have completed a "wall sweep" and should then work together and check all items in the middle of the room up to the selected hip height. Don't forget to check the floor under the rugs. This first searching sweep should also include those items which may be mounted on or in the walls, such as air-conditioning ducts, baseboard heaters, built-in wall cupboards, etc., if these fixtures are below hip height. The first searching sweep usually consumes the most time and effort. During all searching sweeps, use the electronic or medical stethoscope on walls, furniture items, floors, etc.

Second Room Searching Sweep

The man in charge again looks at the furniture or objects in the room and determines the height of the second searching sweep. This height is usually from the hip to the chin or top of the head. The two men return to the starting point and repeat the searching techniques at the second selected searching height. This sweep usually covers pictures hanging on the walls, built-in bookcases, tall table lamps, etc.

Third Room Searching Sweep

When the second searching sweep is completed, the man in charge again determines the next searching height, usually from the chin or the top of the head up to the ceiling. The third sweep is then made. This sweep usually covers

high mounted air-conditioning ducts, hanging light fixtures, etc.

Fourth Room Searching Sweep

If the room has a false or suspended ceiling, the fourth sweep involves investigation of this area. Check flush or ceiling-mounted light fixtures, air-conditioning or ventilation ducts, sound or speaker systems, electrical wiring, structural frame members, etc.

Have a sign or marker posted indicating "Search Completed" conspicuously in the area. Use a piece of colored scotch tape across the door and door jamb approximately two feet above floor level if the use of signs is not practical.

The room searching technique can be expanded. The same basic technique can be used to search a convention hall or airport terminal.

Restated, to search an area you should:

1
Divide the area and select a search height
2
Start from the bottom and work up
3
Start back-to-back and work toward each other
4
Go around the walls then into the center of the room.

Encourage the use of common sense or logic in searching. If a guest speaker at a convention has been threatened, common sense would indicate searching the speakers platform and microphones first, but always return to the searching technique. Do not rely on random or spot checking of only logical target areas. The bomber may not be a logical person.

(For comparison of search systems, see the chart on page 127.)

Suspicious Object Located

Note: It is imperative that personnel involved in the search be instructed that their mission is only to search for and report· suspicious objects, not to move, jar or touch the object or anything attached thereto. The removal/disarming of a bomb must be left to the professionals in explosive ordnance disposal. Remember that bombs and explosives are made to explode, and there are no absolutely safe methods of handling them.

(1) Report the location and an accurate description of the object to the appropriate warden. This information is relayed immediately to the control center who will call police, fire department, and rescue squad. These officers should be met and escorted to the scene.

(2) Place sandbags or mattresses, not metal shield plates, around the object. Do not attempt to cover the object.

(3) Identify the danger area, and b'ock it off with a clear zone of at least 300 feet—include area below and above the object.

(4) Check to see that all doors and windows are open to minimize primary damage from blast and secondary damage from fragmentation.

(5) Evacuate the building.

(6) Do not permit re-entry into the building until the device has been removed/disarmed, and the building declared safe for re-entry.

We in ATF recognize your responsibility to the public and the necessity for maintaining good public relations. This responsibility also includes the safety and protection of the public. We may well be approaching the point, when in the interest of security and protection of people, some inconvenience may have to be imposed on persons visiting public buildings.

Perhaps entrances and exits can be modified with a minimal expenditure to channel all personnel through someone at a registration desk. Personnel entering the building would be required to sign a register showing the name and room number of the person whom they wish to visit. Employees at these regis-

tration desks could contact the person to be visited and advise him that a visitor, by name, is in the lobby. The person to be visited may, in the interest of security and protection, decide to come to the lobby to meet this individual to ascertain that the purpose of the visit is valid and official. A system for signing out when the individual departs could be integrated into this procedure. There is no question that such a procedure would result in many complaints from the public. If it were explained to the visitor by the person at the registration desk that these procedures were implemented in his best interest and safety, the complaints would be reduced.

Other factors for consideration include:

1
Installation of closed-circuit television.

2
Installation of metal detecting devices.

3
Posting of signs indicating the use of closed circuit television or other detection devices.

The above are suggestions—in the final analysis of this entire complex problem, the decision is yours.

Buildings—Their Problem

The physical construction of buildings and their surrounding areas vary widely. Following are a few of the problems search teams will encounter.

Outside Areas

When you search outside areas, pay particular attention to street drainage systems, manholes in the street and in the sidewalk. Thoroughly check trash receptacles, garbage cans, dumpsters, incinerators, etc. Check parked cars and trucks. Check mail boxes if there is a history of placement in your area.

Schools

School bombings are usually directed against non-student areas. Find out which teachers or staff members are unpopular and where they work. The problem areas in schools are student lockers and the chemistry laboratory.

Student lockers are locked; no accurate record of the combinations are available because students change lockers at will. Every other locker seems to "tick." Alarm clocks, wrist watches, leaking thermos jugs and white mice, all make "ticking" sounds. Have the school authorities or police cut off the locks; then search teams should open the lockers. If you cut off the lock you may end up paying for it.

Chemistry labs should be treated with caution. Each year some student tries to make an explosive mixture or rocket fuel in the classroom, gets scared, and phones in a bomb call. The best procedure is to get the chemistry teacher and ask him to inspect the classroom, lab and chemical storage area with you. He will know 90% of the items in the lab which leaves only 10% to worry about.

If repeated bomb threats are received at schools in your area, recommend that the school board hold make-up classes on Saturday. This tends to cut down the number of bomb scares.

Office Buildings

The biggest problem in office buildings is many locked desks. A repair of desk locks is an expensive item. There will be many other items to keep you busy, such as filing cabinets, storage closets, wall lockers, etc. Watch out for the company's security system if they deal in fashions of any type, the automotive or aircraft industry, defense contracts, or the toy industry. Electrical leads, electrical tapes, electrical eyes, electrical pressure mats, electrical microswitches, will all ring those huge bells that no one knows how to turn off.

Auditoriums, Amphitheaters, and Convention Halls

Here, thousands of seats must be checked on hands and knees. Look for cut or unfastened seats with a bomb inserted into the cushion or back. Check out the stage area which has tons of equipment in it; also the speaker's platform and the microphones. The area under the stage generally has crawlways, tunnels, trapdoors, dressing rooms, and storage areas. The sound system is extensive and the air-conditioning system is unbelievable. The entire roof area, in a theater, frequently has one huge storage room and maintenance area above it. Check all hanging decorations and lighting fixtures.

Airport Terminals

This structure combines all problems covered under schools, office buildings, and auditoriums, plus outside areas and aircraft.

AIRCRAFT

The complexities of aircraft design make it unlikely that even the trained searcher will locate any but the most obvious explosive or incendiary device. Thus, detailed searches of large aircraft must be conducted by maintenance and crew personnel who are entirely familiar with the construction and equipment of the plane. In emergency situations where searches must be conducted by public safety personnel without the aid of aircraft specialists, the following general procedures should be used:

1. Evacuate the area and remove all personal property.
2. Check the area around the craft for bombs, wires or evidence of tampering.
3. Tow the aircraft to a distant area.
4. Starting on the outside, work toward the plane's interior.
5. Begin searching at the lowest level and work up.

6. Remove freight and baggage and search cargo areas.

7 Check out rest rooms and lounges.

8. Be alert for small charges placed to rupture the pressure hull or cut control cables. The control cables usually run underneath the center aisle.

9. With special attention to refuse disposal containers, check food preparation and service areas.

10. Search large cabin areas in two sweeps.

11. Check the flight deck.

12. Simultaneously, search the baggage and freight in a safe area under the supervision of airline personnel. If passengers are asked to come forward to identify and open their baggage for inspection, it may be possible to quickly focus in upon unclaimed baggage.

Elevator Wells and Shafts

Elevator wells are usually one to three feet deep with grease, dirt and trash and must be probed by hand. To check elevator shafts, get on the top of the car with two six-volt lanterns, move the car up a floor (or part of a floor) at a time and look around the shaft. Be prepared to find nooks, closets, storage rooms, false panels, walk areas, and hundreds of empty whiskey bottles in paper bags. Don't forget that as you go up, the counterweights are coming down—check them too. The elevator machinery is generally located on the roof. A Word of Caution: Watch for strong winds in the elevator shaft. Don't stand near the edge of the car.

Handling of the News Media

It is of paramount importance that all inquiries by the news media be directed to one person appointed as spokesman. All other persons should be instructed not to discuss the situation with outsiders, especially the news media.

The purpose of this provision is to furnish the news media with accurate information and see that additional bomb threat calls are not precipitated by irresponsible statements from uninformed sources.

Additional Information

Both government and private sources have aids dealing with bomb threats and bombings. Among those available on request from the Bureau of Alcohol, Tobacco and Firearms, Washington, D. C. 20226 are the following:

1. A pamphlet explaining Title XI of the Omnibus Crime Control and Safe Streets Act

2. A booklet of Questions and Answers on Federal Law concerning explosives under Title XI

3. A reprint of Title XI of the Law

"Property Protection During Civil Disturbances" is available from Factory Insurance Association, 85 Woodland St., Hartford, Connecticut 06102.

The publishing house of Charles C. Thomas, 301 East Lawrence Ave., Springfield, Illinois 62717, has four books on the subject: "Explosives and Homemade Bombs" by Stoffel; "Bombs and Bombings" by Tom G. Brodie; "Explosives and Bomb Disposal Guide" by Lenz; and "Protection Against Bombs and Incendiaries" by Pike.

Three films entitled "Bombs I, II and III" are available from Motorola Tele- programs, Inc., Suite 26, 4825 N. Scott St., Schiller Park, Ilinois 60176, ATTN: Mr. Lloyd Singer, President. These are on 16 mm, Super 8 mm, Videotape and Videocasettes. They also have a work- book on bomb scare planning and con- duct seminars. Mail your request for information on a company letterhead.

William Brose Productions Inc., 3168 Oakshire Drive, Hollywood, California 90068, has two films: "Bomb Threat! Plan Don't Panic" (15 min.); and "High- fire! Plan for Survival" (19 min.) The last deals with evacuating high rise office buildings.

LETTER AND PACKAGE BOMBS

Background

Letter and package bombs are not new. While the latest incidents have involved political terrorism, such bombs are made for a wide variety of mo- tives. The particular form of these bombs varies in size, shape and com- ponents. They may have electric, nonelectric or other sophisticated firing systems.

Precautions

Mail handlers should be alert to recognize suspicious looking items. Mail should be separated into "personal" and "business". Although there is no approved, standard detection method, the following precautions are sug- gested:

a. Look at the sender's address. Is it a familiar one?

b. Is correspondence from the sender expected?
   Do the characteristics of the envelope or package resemble the ex- pected contents?

c. If the item is from another country, ask yourself if it is expected. Do you have relatives or friends traveling? Did you buy something from business associates, charitable or religious groups, internation- al organizations, etc.?

IF YOU HAVE A SUSPICIOUS LOOKING LETTER OR PACKAGE:

DO NOT TRY TO OPEN IT.

ISOLATE IT AND EVACUATE EVERYONE IN THE VICINITY TO A SAFE DISTANCE.

NOTIFY LOCAL POLICE AND AWAIT THEIR ARRIVAL.

Suggested form to be completed by investigators following

BOMB
THREAT
CALLS

Type of Complainant:

☐ School   ☐ Hospital   ☐ Industrial Manufacturing Company   ☐ Business
☐ Other

Business Name of Complainant

Business Address

Business Telephone

Name of Person Reporting Complaint

Telephone Number That Call Was Received On   Date and Time of Call

Name of Person Who Talked to the Caller

Exact Words said by Caller

Background Noises (i.e., Street Sounds, Baby Crying, etc.)

Information about Caller:

Age   Sex   Race   Accent   Educational Level

Speech Impediments (Drunk, Lisp, etc.)   Attitude (Calm, Excited, etc.)

Any Suspects?
☐ Yes   ☐ No

Have Previous Calls Been Received?   If Yes, Approximately How Many?
☐ Yes   ☐ No

Has the Telephone Company Security Department Been Notified?
☐ Yes   ☐ No

Was any Incendiary or Explosive Device Found?
☐ Yes   ☐ No

Number of Threats Received Thus Far During Calendar Year

CHECK LIST WHEN YOU RECEIVE A BOMB THREAT

Time and Date Reported: _____

How Reported: _____

Exact Words of Caller: _____

_____

_____

Questions to Ask: _____

1. When is bomb going to explode? _____

2. Where is bomb right now? _____

3. What kind of bomb is it? _____

4. What does it look like? _____

5. Why did you place the bomb? _____

6. Where are you calling from? _____

Description of Callers Voice: _____

Male _____ Female _____ Young _____ Middle Age _____ Old _____ Accent _____

Tone of Voice _____ Background Noise _____ Is voice familiar? _____

If so, who did it sound like? _____

_____

Other voice characteristics: _____

Time Caller Hung Up: _____ Remarks: _____

_____

_____

_____

Name, Address, Telephone of Recipient: _____

_____

_____

RECORD:

1. Date _____ and time _____ of call.

2. Exact language used. _____
   _____
   _____
   _____
   _____
   _____
   _____

3. ☐ Male   ☐ Female
   ☐ Adult   ☐ Child
   Estimated age _____ Race _____

4. Speech (Check applicable boxes)

   ☐ Slow   ☐ Excited   ☐ Disguised
   ☐ Rapid   ☐ Loud   ☐ Broken
   ☐ Normal   ☐ Normal   ☐ Sincere

   Accent _____

5. Background noises _____
   _____
   _____
   _____
   _____
   _____

6. Name of person receiving the call

SEARCH SYSTEMS

	ADVANTAGES	DISADVANTAGES	THOROUGHNESS
SUPERVISORY **SEARCH BY: Supervisors** BEST for Covert search POOR for thoroughness POOR for morale if detected	1. Covert 2. Fairly rapid 3. Loss of working time of supervisor only	1. Unfamiliarity with many areas. 2. Will not look in dirty places 3. Covert search is difficult to maintain 4. Generally results in search of obvious areas, *not* hard-to-reach ones 5. Violation of privacy problems 6. Danger to unevacuated workers	50-65%
OCCUPANT **SEARCH BY: Occupants** BEST for speed of search GOOD for thoroughness GOOD for morale (with confidence in training given beforehand)	1. Rapid 2. No privacy violation problem 3. Loss of work time for shorter period of time than for evacuation 4. Personal concern for own safety leads to good search 5. Personnel conducting search are familiar with area	1. Requires training of entire work force 2. Requires several practical training exercises 3. Danger to unevacuated workers	80-90%
TEAM **SEARCH BY: Trained Team** BEST for safety BEST for thoroughness BEST for morale POOR for lost work time	1. Thorough 2. No danger to workers who have been evacuated 3. Workers feel company cares for their safety	1. Loss of production time 2. Very slow operation 3. Requires comprehensive training and practice 4. Privacy violation problems	90-100%

General Information from the Controlled Substances Inventory List[*]

―――――

*Prepared by the U.S. Department of Justice, Drug Enforcement Administration, Washington, D.C. 20537. Reprinted with permission.

INVENTORY REQUIREMENTS

The Controlled Substances Act (P.L. 91-513) requires each registrant to make a complete and accurate record of all stocks of controlled substances on hand every two years. The biennial inventory date of May 1, may be changed by the registrant to fit his regular general physical inventory date, if any, so long as the date is not more than six (6) months from the biennial date that would otherwise apply. The actual taking of the inventory should not vary more than four (4) days from the biennial inventory date.

Whether or not you use this inventory format, the inventory record must:

1. list the name, address, and DEA registration number of the registrant.
2. indicate the date and the time the inventory is taken, i.e., opening or close of business.
3. be signed by the person or persons responsible for taking the inventory.
4. be maintained at the location appearing on the registration certificate for at least two years.
5. keep records of Schedule II drugs separate from all other controlled substances.

When taking the inventory of Schedule II controlled substances, an exact count or measure must be made. When taking the inventory of Schedule III, IV, and V, controlled substances, an estimated count may be made unless the container holds more than 1,000 dosage units, in which case an exact count must be made if the container has been opened.

GENERAL INFORMATION

FOR PHARMACISTS

Schedules of Controlled Substances

The Drugs that come under jurisdiction of the Controlled Substances Act are divided into five Schedules. They are as follows:

Schedule I Substances

Drugs in this schedule are those that have no accepted medical use in the United States and have a high abuse potential. Some examples are heroin, marihuana, LSD, peyote, mescaline, psilocybin, tetrahydrocannabinols, ketobemidone, levomoramide, racemoramide, benzylmorphine, dihydromorphine, morphine, methysulfonate, nicocodeine, nicomorphine, etorphine, and others.

Schedule II Substances

The drugs in this schedule have a high abuse potential with severe psychic or physical dependence liability. Examples of Schedule II controlled substances are certain narcotic drugs, and drugs containing amphetamines or methamphetamines as the single active ingredient, or in combination with each other. Additional examples of Schedule II controlled substances are: opium, morphine, codeine, hydromorphone (Dilaudid), methadone (Dolophine), pantopon, meperidine (Demerol), cocaine, oxycodone (Percodan), anileridine (Leritine), oxymorphone (Numorphan); and amphetamine (Benzedrine, Dexedrine) and methamphetamine (Desoxyn). Also in Schedule II are phenmetrazine (Preludin), methylphenidate (Ritalin), amobarbital, pentobarbital, secobarbital, methaqualone, etorphine HCl, and dyphenoxylate.

Schedule III Substances

The drugs in this schedule have an abuse potential less than those in Schedules I and II, and include compounds containing limited quantities of certain narcotic drugs, and non-narcotic drugs such as: derivatives of barbituric acid except those that are listed in another Schedule, glutethimide (Doriden), methyprylon (Noludar), chlorhexadol, phencyclidine, sulfondiethylmethane, sulfonmethane, nalorphine, benzphetamine, chlorphentermine, clortermine, mazindol, phendimetrazine. Paregoric is in this Schedule.

Schedule IV Substances

The drugs in this schedule have an abuse potential less than those listed in Schedule III and include such drugs as: barbital, phenobarbital, methylphenobarbital, chloral betaine (Beta Chlor), chloral hydrate, ethchlorvynol (Placidyl), ethinamate (Valmid), meprobamate (Equanil, Miltown), paraldehyde, methodexital, fenfluramine, diethylpropion, phentermine, chlordiazepoxide (Librium), diazepam (Valium), oxazepam (Serax), clorazepate (Tranxene), flurazepam (Dalmane), clanazepam, and mebutamate.

Schedule V Substances

The drugs in this schedule have an abuse potential less than those listed in Schedule IV and consist of preparations containing limited quantities of certain narcotic drugs generally for antitussive and antidiarrheal purposes. which may be distributed without a prescription order.

Retail Distribution Restrictions For Schedule V Substances

Schedule V controlled substances or any controlled substance which is not a prescription item under the Federal Food, Drug, and Cosmetic Act, may be distributed without a prescription order at retail provided that:

1) Such distribution is made only by a pharmacist and not by a non-pharmacist employee even if under the direct supervision of a pharmacist. However, after the pharmacist has fulfilled his professional and legal responsibilities, the actual cash, credit transaction, or delivery, may be completed by a non-pharmacist.

2) Not more than 240 ml. (8 fluid ounces) or not more than 48 solid dosage units of any substance containing opium, nor more than 120 ml. (4 fluid ounces) or not more than 24 solid dosage units of any other controlled substance, may be distributed at retail to the same purchaser in any given 48-hour period without a valid prescription order.

3) The purchaser at retail is at least 18 years of age.

4) The pharmacist requires every purchaser at retail of a Schedule V controlled substance not known to him to furnish suitable identification (including proof of age where appropriate).

5) A Schedule V bound record book is maintained which contains the name and address of the purchaser, kind and quantity of controlled substance purchased, date of each sale and initials of the dispensing pharmacist. This record book shall be maintained for a period of two years from the date of the last transaction entered in such record book, and it shall be made available for inspection and copying by officers of the United States, authorized by the Attorney General.

6) Other Federal, state, or local law does not require a prescription order.

Symbols and Labeling

Each commerical container of controller substances is required to have on its label a symbol designating to which Schedule it belongs. The symbol for Schedule I through V controlled substances is as follows: C or C-1; C or C-II; C or C-III; C or C-IV; and C or C-V. These symbols are not required on prescription containers dispensed by a pharmacist to a patient in the course of his professional practice.

Registration

Every pharmacy engaged in distributing or dispensing any controlled substance must register with the Drug Enforcement Administration. The registration must be renewed annually and the certificate of registration must be maintained at the registered location and kept available for official inspections. If a person owns and operates more than one pharmacy, he must register each place of business. A registration fee of $5.00 is charged annually for each registration. Every pharmacy will receive a re-registration application approximately 60 days before the expiration date of his registration each year. If a registered pharmacy does not receive such forms within 45 days before the expiration date of his registration; he must give notice of such fact and request the re-registration forms by writing to the Registration Section of the Drug Enforcement Administration.

New Registrations

Pharmacies that seek to become registered for the first time must request a registration application for new registrants from the Drug Enforcement Administration, P.O. Box 28083, Central Station, Washington, D.C. 2005, or from any DEA Regional Office. Modifications such as change of address, location, or name by existing registrants may be made in accordance with § 1301.61, Title 21, code of Federal Regulations.

Any pharmacy engaged in co-op buying of controlled substances must register as a distributor with the Drug Enforcement Administration.

In order to be registered as a distributor, a pharmacy must meet the security requirements as set forth for a distributor (wholesaler) and keep records required of a distributor.

Records

Every pharmacy engaged in handling of controlled substances must keep complete and accurate records of all receiving and dispensing transactions. All such records shall be maintained for a period of two years.

All inventories and records of controlled substances in Schedule II must be maintained separately from all other records of the registrant. All inventories and records of controlled substances in Schedules III, IV, and V must be maintained separately or must be in such form that they are readily retrievable from the ordinary professional and business records of the pharmacy.

All records pertaining to controlled substances shall be made available for inspection and copying by duly authorized officials of the Drug Enforcement Administration.

When a registrant first engages in business, and every two years thereafter, he must make a complete and accurate inventory of all stocks of controlled substances on hand. This inventory record shall be kept by the registrant for a period of two years. *Pharmacies are not required to submit a copy of the inventory to the Drug Enforcement Administration.*

Continuing Records to be Kept by a Pharmacy

Every pharmacy must maintain on a current basis a complete and accurate record of each controlled substance received.

Copy 3 of executed Order Forms retained by the pharmacy which have been completed as described under section entitled: "Order Forms" will constitute a pharmacy's receiving records for Schedule II controlled substances. Invoices for Schedules III, IV, and V controlled substances will be considered as complete receiving records *if the actual date of receipt is clearly recorded on the invoices by the pharmacist or other responsible individual.*

Order Forms

A triplicate order form is necessary for the transfer of controlled substances in Schedules I and II. Under the Controlled Substances Act, the use of the order forms will be for Schedules I and II drugs only. A registrant desiring DEA order forms can obtain them by using the requisition form (DEA-222D). Once a registrant has obtained DEA order forms, they will then utilize Form DEA-222B which is in each order form book. No charge is made for order forms.

When a registrant issues an order form for Schedule II controlled substances and when he receives the items ordered he must record, on his retained copy, the number of packages and the date such packages were received. A space is provided for this on the DEA order form.

DEA order form books consist of six sets of order forms. Each pharmacy is allowed a maximum of three books at one time unless it can show that its needs exceed this limit. In such case, the pharmacy should contact the Regional Office of DEA in its area and explain its needs.

Lost or Stolen Order Forms

Lost or stolen order forms should not be reported to the Registration Section of DEA. Instead, direct your information to: Drug Enforcement Administration, Compliance Division, Investigations Section, 1405 I Street, N.W., Washington, D.C. 20537.

Prescription Orders

Prescription orders that are dispensed for controlled substances in Schedule II must be typewritten, written in ink, or indelible pencil and must be signed by the practitioner issuing such prescription orders.

No prescription order for a controlled substance in Schedule II may be refilled and such prescription orders must be kept in a separate file.

Prescription orders for controlled substances in Schedules III, IV, or V may be issued either orally or in writing from a practitioner and may be re-dispensed if so authorized. Such prescription orders may not be dispensed or re-dispensed more than six months after the date issued, or be refilled more than five times after the date issued. If a physician wishes a patient to continue on the medication a new prescription order is required. Oral prescription orders must be promptly committed to writing and filed by the pharmacist.

The label of any drug listed as a "controlled substance" in Schedules II, III, or IV of the Controlled Substances Act shall, when dispensed to or for a patient, contain the following warning:

> CAUTION: "Federal law prohibits the transfer of this drug to any person other than the patient for whom it was prescribed."

A pharmacist after refilling a prescription order for any controlled substance in Schedules III, IV, or V, must enter on the back of that prescription order his initials, the date such prescription order was refilled, and the amount of drug dispensed on such refill. If the pharmacist merely initials and dates the back of the prescription order he shall be deemed to have dispensed a refill for the full face amount of the original prescription order.

The partial dispensing of a Schedule II controlled substance* is permissible, if the pharmacist is unable to supply the full quantity called for in a written or emergency oral prescription order. He may supply a portion of the quantity requested provided he makes a notation of the quantity supplied on the face of the written prescription order (or written record of the emergency oral prescription) and so advises the authorizing practitioner. The remaining portion may be dispensed within 72 hours of the first dispensing. No further quantity may be supplied beyond the 72 hours except on a new prescription order.

Partial Dispensing of Schedules III and IV Controlled Substance Prescription Orders*

Partial dispensing of prescription orders for controlled substances in Schedules III and IV is permitted if the pharmacist dispensing or refilling the prescription order sets forth the quantity dispensed and his initials on the back of the prescription order. In addition, the partial dispensing may not exceed the total amount authorized in the prescription order and the dispensing of all refills must be within the six month limit.

Filing of Prescription Orders for Controlled Substances

Prescription orders for controlled substances must be filed in one of the following three ways:

1) A pharmacy can maintain three separate files—a file for Schedule II drugs dispensed, a file for Schedules III, IV, and V drugs dispensed, and a file for prescription orders for all other drugs dispensed.

2) A pharmacy can maintain two files—a file for all Schedule II drugs dispensed and another file for all other drugs dispensed including those in Schedules III, IV, and V. If this method is used, the prescription orders in the file for Schedules III, IV, and V must be stamped with the letter "C" in red ink, not less than one inch high, in the lower right corner. This distinctive marking makes the records "readily retrievable" for inspection.

3) A pharmacy can maintain two files—one file for all controlled drugs in all Schedules and a second file for all prescription orders for non-controlled drugs dispensed. If this method is used, the prescription orders for drugs in Schedules III, IV, and V in the controlled drug prescription file must be stamped with the red letter "C" not less than one inch high in the lower right corner, as previously mentioned.

In states where the Uniform Narcotic Act (or other state law) requires all narcotic prescription records be kept together, DEA is of the opinion that a positive conflict exists between Federal and state law and, under Section 708 of the Controlled Substances Act, Federal requirements prevail.

Emergency Dispensing of Schedule II Controlled Substances

In the case of a bona fide emergency situation, as defined by the Secretary of Health, Education, and Welfare, a pharmacist may dispense a Schedule II controlled substance upon receiving oral authorization of a prescribing practitioner provided that:

---

*Regulations pertaining to the partial dispensing of Schedule II controlled substances to allow for unit dose systems for patients in long term care facilities were under review at the time this publication was being prepared. Consult your local DEA Regional Office for current information.

1) The quantity prescribed and dispensed is limited to the amount adequate to treat the patient during the emergency period. Prescribing or dispensing beyond the emergency period must be pursuant to a written prescription order.

2) The prescription order shall be immediately reduced to writing by the pharmacist and shall contain all information, except for the prescribing practitioner's signature.

3) If the prescribing practitioner is not known to the pharmacist, he must make a reasonable effort to determine that the oral authorization came from a practitioner, by verifying his telephone number against that listed in the directory and other good faith efforts to insure his identity.

4) Within 72 hours after authorizing an emergency oral prescription order, the prescribing practitioner must cause a written prescription order for the emergency quantity prescribed to be delivered to the dispensing pharmacist. The prescription order shall have written on its face "Authorization for Emergency Dispensing." The written prescription order may be delivered in person or by mail, but if delivered by mail it must be postmarked within the 72 hour period. Upon receipt, the dispensing pharmacist shall attach this prescription order to the oral emergency prescription order which had earlier been reduced to writing. *The pharmacist shall notify the nearest office of DEA if the prescribing practitioner fails to deliver a written prescription order to him; failure of the pharmacist to do so shall void the authority conferred by the subsection to dispense without a written prescription order of a prescribing practitioner.*

For the purpose of authorizing an oral prescription order of a controlled substance listed in Schedule II of the Federal Controlled Substances Act, the term "emergency situation" means those situations in which the prescribing practitioner determines that:

1) Immediate administration of the controlled substance is necessary for the proper treatment of the intended ultimate user; and,

2) No appropriate alternative treatment is available, including administration of a drug which is not a controlled substance under Schedule II of the Act; and,

3) It is not reasonably possible for the prescribing practitioner to provide a written prescription order to be presented to the person dispensing the substance, prior to the dispensing.

An emergency means a situation where a quantity of a controlled substance may be dispensed by a pharmacy to a patient who does not have an alternative source for such substance reasonably available to him, and the pharmacy cannot obtain such substances through his normal distribution channels within the time required to meet the immediate needs of the patient for such substance.

Distribution by a Pharmacy

A pharmacy (as well as all practitioner registrants) registered to dispense a controlled substance may distribute (without being registered to distribute) a quantity of such substances to another pharmacy for the purpose of general dispensing by that pharmacy provided that the following conditions are met:

1) The pharmacy to which the controlled substance is being distributed is registered under the Act to dispense that controlled substance.

2) The distribution is recorded as being dispensed by the first pharmacy and the second pharmacy records the substance as being received. Each pharmacy will retain a signed receipt of the distribution.

3) If the substance is listed in Schedule I or II, the transfer must be made on an official order form.

4) The total number of dosage units of controlled substances distributed by a pharmacy may not exceed 5 percent of all controlled substances dispensed by the pharmacy for a 12 month period. If at any time it does exceed 5 percent the pharmacy is required to register as a distributor as well as being registered as a pharmacy.

Drug Security and Control

The following methods of drug security and control are required by the Drug Enforcement Administration:

Security—Pharmacies must keep Schedules II, III, IV, and V controlled substances in a locked cabinet or dispersed throughout the non-controlled stock in such a manner to obstruct theft.

Disposal—A pharmacy wishing to dispose of any excess or undesired stocks of controlled substances must contact his nearest DEA Regional or District Office and request the necessary forms (DEA-41). Three copies of Form DEA-41 will be forwarded to the Regional Office which serves the area in which the pharmacy is situated.

A cover letter from the pharmacy must be attached to the reports stating that the controlled substances are not desired and the pharmacy wishes to dispose of them.

Regional Office Action Upon Receipt of Request to Destroy Controlled Substances.

Upon receipt of the required DEA-41 forms and the letter from the pharmacy, one of four courses of action will be utilized. The course of action chosen by the Regional Director or his designee will be stated in letter form, attached to the original copy of the DEA-41 form, and returned to the pharmacy.

The four courses of action in disposing of excess or undesired stock of controlled substances are:

1) The return letter to the pharmacy will advise that the drugs may be destroyed by two responsible parties employed or acting on behalf of the registrant. This course of action will be used when there are factors which preclude an on-the-site destruction witnessed by DEA personnel, such as the firm's history of compliance and the abuse potential of the drugs involved.

2) The return letter to the pharmacy will advise to forward the excess or undesired stocks or controlled substances to the appropriate state agency for destruction. In lieu of actual surrender to the state agency, destructions witnessed by state personnel are acceptable.

3) The return letter will advise to hold the substances until DEA personnel arrive at a mutually convenient time to witness the destruction of the substances. DEA personnel will date and sign the reports or forms after witnessing the destruction.

4) The return letter will advise to forward the substances to the Regional Office of DEA which serves the area in which the registrant is located. Upon receipt of the substances, the Regional Director or his designee will verify the actual substance submitted. If errors are found, a corrected form must be prepared and the registrant duly notified. The original form will be returned to the registrant.

Drug Theft—Any pharmacy involved in loss of controlled substances must notify the DEA Regional Office in its region of the theft or significant loss upon discovery. The pharmacy must make a report regarding the loss or theft by completing DEA Form 106.

Such report shall contain the following information:

1) Name and address of firm.

2) DEA Registration Number.

3) Date of theft.

4) Local police department notified.

5) Type of theft (night break-in, armed robbery, etc.).

6) Listing of symbols or cost code used by pharmacy in marking containers (if any).

7) Listing of controlled substances missing through theft.

The above report should be made in triplicate. The pharmacy should keep the original copy for its records and forward the remaining two copies to the nearest DEA Regional or District Office.

A Manual for the Medical Practitioner: An Informational Outline of the Controlled Substances Act of 1970 *

*Prepared by the U.S. Department of Justice, Drug Enforcement Administration, Washington, D.C. 20537. Reprinted with permission.

Drug Enforcement Administration

The Drug Enforcement Administration is the lead Federal law enforcement agency charged with the responsibility of combating drug abuse. The Administration was established July 1, 1973 by Presidential Reorganization Plan No. 2 of 1973. It resulted from the merger of the Bureau of Narcotics and Dangerous Drugs, the Office for Drug Abuse Law Enforcement, the Office of National Narcotic Intelligence, those elements of the Bureau of Customs which had drug investigative responsibilites, and those functions of the Office of Science and Technology which were drug enforcement related. The Administration was established to control more effectively narcotic and dangerous drug abuse through enforcement and prevention. In carrying out its mission, the Administration cooperates with other Federal agencies, foreign as well as State and local governments, private industry, and other organizations.

Since 1914, the Congress has enacted more than 50 pieces of legislation relating to control and diversion of drugs. The Controlled Substances Act of 1970 became effective May 1, 1971. It collects and conforms most of these diverse laws into one piece of legislation. The law is designed to improve the administration and regulation of manufacturing, distribution, and the dispensing of Controlled Substances by providing a "closed" system for legitimate handlers of these drugs. Such a closed system should help reduce the widespread diversion of these drugs out of legitimate channels that find their way into the illicit market.

This informational outline has been prepared to acquaint the physician with requirements set up under the Controlled Substances Act of 1970, as they affect various classes of practitioners.

The drugs and drug products that come under the jurisdiction of the Controlled Substances Act are divided into five Schedules. Some examples in each Schedule are outlined below. For a complete listing of all the controlled drugs, contact any Regional Office of the Drug Enforcement Administration. The addresses are listed in the back portion of this outline.

NOTE: The "physician" as used in this booklet, means any physician, dentist, podiatrist, veterinarian, or other practitioner authorized to administer, dispense, and prescribe Controlled Substances.

Schedules of Controlled Drugs

The drugs that come under jurisdiction of the Controlled Substances Act are divided into five schedules. They are as follows:

Schedule I Substances
Drugs in this schedule are those that have no accepted medical use in the United States and have a high abuse potential. Some examples are Heroin, Marihuana, LSD, Peyote, Mescaline, Psilocybin, Tetrahydrocannabinols, Ketobemidone, Levomoramide, Racemoramide, Benzylmorphine, Dihydromorphine, Morphine methylsulfonate, Nicocodeine, Nicomorphine, and others.

Schedule II Substances
The drugs in this schedule have a high abuse potential with severe psychic or physical dependence liability. Schedule II controlled substances consist of certain narcotic drugs, and drugs containing amphetamines or methamphetamines as the single active ingredient, or in combination with each other. Examples of Schedule II controlled substances are: opium, morphine, codeine, hydromorphone (Dilaudid), methadone (Dolophine), Pantopon, Meperdine (Demerol), Cocaine, Oxycodone (Percodan), Anileridine (Leritine), Oxymorphone (Numorphan); and straight Amphetamines and Methamphetamines. Also in Schedule II are Phenmetrazine (Preludin), Methylphenidate (Ritalin), Amobarbital, Pentobarbital, Secobarbital, and Methaqualone.

Schedule III Substances
The drugs in this schedule have an abuse potential less than those in Schedules I and II, and include compounds containing limited quantities of certain narcotic drugs, and non-narcotic drugs such as: derivatives of barbituric acid except those that are listed in another Schedule, Glutethimide (Doriden), Methyprylon (Noludar), Chlorhexadol, Phencyclidine, Sulfondiethylmethane, Sulfonmenthane, Nalorphine, Benzphetamine, Chlorphentermine, Clortermine, Mazindol, Phendimetrazine. Paregoric is in this Schedule.

Schedule IV Substances
The drugs in this schedule have an abuse potential less than those listed in Schedule III and include such drugs as: Barbital, Phenobarbital, Methylphenobarbital, Chloral Betaine (Beta Chlor), Chloral Hydrate, Ethchlorvynol (Placidyl), Ethinamate (Valmid), Meprobamate (Equanil, Miltown), Paraldehyde, Pentaerythritol Chloral (Petrichloral) Methohexital, Fenfluramine, Diethylpropion, Phentermine, Chlordiazepoxide (Librium), Diazepam (Valium), Oxazepam (Serax), Clorazepate (Tranxene), Flurazepam (Dalmane), and Clanazepam.

Schedule V Substances
The drugs in this schedule have an abuse potential less than those listed in Schedule IV and consist of preparations containing moderate, limited quantities of certain narcotic drugs generally for antitussive and antidiarrheal purposes, which may be distributed without a prescription order.

Application of State Law and Federal Law

Nothing in this pamphlet shall be construed as authorizing or permitting any person to do any act which he is not authorized or permitted to do under other Federal or State laws. In addition, none of the policy and information in this pamphlet may be construed as authorizing or permitting any person to do any act which he is not authorized, or refuse to meet any requirements imposed under the regulations published in the most recent publication of Title 21, Chapter II, of the Federal Register.

Registration of Practitioners

Every physician who administers, prescribes, or dispenses any of the drugs listed in the five Schedules must be registered with the Drug Enforcement Administration.

"Administer" means to instill a drug into the body of the patient.

"Prescribe" means to issue a prescription for the patient.

"Dispense" means the giving of drugs in some type of bottle, box or other container to the patient.

(*Under the act, the definition of "dispense" also includes the administering of Controlled Substances.*)

Physicians are required to register with the Drug Enforcement Administration, Registration Section, P.O. Box 28083, Central Station, Washington, D.C. 20005. A physician who seeks to become registered must apply on Form DEA-224, which can be obtained from the Registration Section or from any DEA Regional Office. Complete instructions accompany the form.

If a physician has more than one office in which he administers and/or dispenses any of the drugs listed in the five Schedules, he then is required to register at each office. However, if a physician only administers and/or dispenses at his principal office and only writes prescription orders at the other office or offices, he then is only required to register at his principal office where he administers and/or dispenses, provided each office is within the same state.

The registration fee is $5.00 annually for each place of registration.

Sample Form DEA-224

Below is a sample format of a completed Form DEA-224. Attention should be paid to Item (2) as triplicate order forms will not be issued unless the appropriate drug schedules are checked.

Registration Regarding Interns, Residents, and Foreign Physicians

Any physician who is an intern, resident, or foreign physician may dispense, administer, and prescribe controlled drugs under the registration of a hospital or other institution which is registered and by whom the physician is employed, provided that:

1. The dispensing, administering, or prescribing is in the usual course of his professional practice;
2. The physician is authorized or permitted to do so by the jurisdiction in which he is practicing;
3. The hospital or institution has verified that the physician is permitted to dispense, administer, or prescribe drugs within the jurisdiction;
4. The physician acts only within the scope of his employment in the hospital or institution;
5. The hospital or institution authorizes the intern, resident, or foreign physician to dispense or prescribe under its registration and assigns a specific code number for each physician so authorized. An example of code number is as follows:

DEA Registration   AB1234567-012   Hospital Code
Number   Number

6. A current list of internal codes and the corresponding individual practitioners is kept by the hospital or other institution and is made available at all times to other registrants and law enforcement agencies upon request for the purpose of verifying the authority of the prescribing individual practitioner.

Records

In order for the Drug Enforcement Administration to curtail the diversion of controlled drugs, it is necessary for manufacturers, wholesalers, pharmacies, hospitals, and certain physicians, among others, to keep records of drugs purchased, distributed, and dispensed. Having this closed system, a controlled drug can be traced from the time it was manufactured to the time it was dispensed to the ultimate user.

Narcotic Drugs

A physician who *prescribes* and/or *administers* narcotic drugs in the lawful course of his professional practice is *not* required to keep records of those transactions. If a physician *dispenses* a narcotic drug to a patient, he *is* required to keep a record of such dispensing.

Non-Narcotic Drugs

A physician who regularly engages in dispensing any of the non-narcotic drugs listed in the Schedules to his patients *as a regular part of his professional practice*, and for which he charges his patients either separately or together with other professional services, must keep records of all such drugs received and dispensed. The records must be kept for a period of two years and are subject to inspection by the Drug Enforcement Administration. (*Dispensed as used above includes administering.*)

A physician who occasionally dispenses a non-narcotic controlled drug to a patient (such as a physician's sample) is not required to maintain records of such dispensing.

Inventory

A physician who regularly engages in dispensing drugs and is required to keep records as stated above must take an inventory every two years of all stocks of controlled drugs on hand. A physician who plans to dispense drugs regularly, is requested to take the initial inventory when he first engages in dispensing. A physician must keep this record for two years and is *not* required to submit a copy to the DEA.

Order Forms

A physician who has need for controlled drugs in Schedule II for use in his office or medical bag, must obtain these drugs by the use of a triplicate order form. Order forms can be obtained from the Drug Enforcement Administration, Registration Section, P.O. Box 28083, Central Station, Washington, D.C. 20005, by using the requisition Form DEA-222D. Once a physician has obtained the new DEA order forms, he will then utilize Form DEA-222B which is found in each order form book.

The Federal Triplicate Order Forms should not be confused with the triplicate prescription blanks that are required by some states. The Federal order forms are to be used by a physician when he has a need for a drug in Schedule II which is to be used in his office. For example, a physician must fill out a Triplicate Order Form in order to obtain Demerol or Morphine, etc. from his normal source of supply.

Sample Order Form

Below is a sample format of a completed order form.

For instructions on completing and executing order forms, see the inside front cover of the Order Form Book.

Prescription Orders

Who May Issue

A prescription order for a controlled substance may be issued only by a physician, dentist, podiatrist, veterinarian, or other registered practitioner who is:

(1) Authorized to prescribe controlled substances by the jurisdiction in which he is licensed to practice his profession; and

(2) Either registered under the Controlled Substances Act or exempted from registration (military and Public Health Service physicians).

Execution of Prescription Orders by Physicians

All prescription orders for controlled substances shall be dated as of, and signed on, the date when issued and must bear the full name and address of the patient, and the name, address, and registration number of the physician. Where an oral order is not permitted, prescription orders must be written in ink or indelible pencil or typewriter and must be manually signed by the practitioner. The prescription orders may be prepared by a nurse or secretary for the signature of the physician, but the prescribing physician is responsible in case the prescription order does not conform in all essential respects to the law and regulations.

A written prescription order is required for drugs in Schedule II and must be signed by the physician. The refilling of Schedule II prescription orders is prohibited.

A prescription order for drugs in Schedules III, IV, and V may be issued either orally or in writing and may be renewed if so authorized on the prescription. However, the prescription order may only be renewed up to five times within six months after the date of issue. After five renewals or after six months, a new prescription order is required either orally or in writing from the physician.

Emergency Telephone Prescription Order for Schedule II Drugs

In the case of a bonafide emergency, a physician may telephone a prescription order to a pharmacist for a drug in Schedule II. In such a case, the drug prescribed must be limited to the amount needed to treat his patient during the emergency period. The physician must furnish, within 72 hours, a written, signed prescription order to the pharmacy for the drug prescribed. The pharmacist is required by law to notify DEA if he has not received the written prescription order within the 72 hours.

"Emergency" means that the immediate administration of the drug is necessary for proper treatment, that no alternative treatment is available and it is not possible for the physician to provide a written prescription order for the drug at that time.

Discontinuance of Practice by a Physician

A physician who discontinues his practice must return his Registration Certificate and any unused order forms to the nearest office of the DEA. A physician having Controlled Substances in his possession at the time of discontinuing practice should obtain information from the Regional Office of the DEA in his area on how to dispose of these drugs.

Security

A physician who has Controlled Substances stored in his office or clinic must keep these drugs in a securely locked, substantially constructed cabinet or safe.

Drug Theft

A physician involved in the loss of Controlled Drugs by theft must notify the Regional Office of the DEA in his area at the time the theft is discovered. The Regional Office will provide information on what reports are required of the physician. The physician should also notify his local police department of such theft.

DEA Domestic Regional Offices

Region I—Boston
JFK Federal Building, Room G-64
Boston, Massachusetts 02203
(617) 223-2170
(Connecticut, Maine,
Massachusetts, New Hampshire,
Rhode Island, Vermont)

Region II—New York
555 West 57th Street
Suite 1900
New York, New York 10019
(212) 660-5151
(New York, Northern New Jersey)

Region III—Philadelphia
William J. Green Federal Building
600 Arch Street
Room 10224
Philadelphia, Pennsylvania 19106
(215) 597-9530
(Delaware, Southern New Jersey,
Pennsylvania)

Region IV—Baltimore
31 Hopkins Plaza, Room 955
Baltimore, Maryland 21201
(301) 962-4800
(District of Columbia,
Maryland, North Carolina,
Virginia, West Virginia)

Region V—Miami
8400 N.W. 53rd Street
Miami, Florida 33166
(305) 350-4451
(Florida, Georgia, South
Carolina, Puerto Rico)

Region VI—Detroit
357 Federal Building and
U.S. Courthouse
231 West Lafayette
Detroit, Michigan 48226
(313) 226-7290
(Kentucky, Michigan, Ohio)

Region VII—Chicago
1800 Dirksen Federal Building
219 South Dearborn Street
Chicago, Illinois 60604
(312) 353-7875
(Illinois, Indiana, Wisconsin)

Region VIII—New Orleans
1001 Howard Avenue
Suite 1800 Plaza Tower
New Orleans, Louisiana 70113
(504) 589-6841
(Alabama, Arkansas,
Louisiana, Mississippi,
Tennessee)

Region X—Kansas City
U.S. Courthouse, Suite 231
811 Grand Avenue
Kansas City, Missouri 64106
(816) 374-2631
(Minnesota, North Dakota,
South Dakota, Iowa, Kansas,
Missouri, Nebraska)

Region XI—Dallas
Earle Cabell Federal Building
1100 Commerce Street
Room 4A5
Dallas, Texas 75202
(214) 749-3631
(Oklahoma, Texas)

Region XII—Denver
U.S. Custom House
Room 336, P.O. Box 1860
Denver, Colorado 80201
(303) 837-3951
(Arizona, Colorado, New Mexico,
Utah, Wyoming)

Region XIII—Seattle
U.S. Courthouse
221 First Avenue West
Room 200
Seattle, Washington 98119
(206) 442-5443
(Alaska, Idaho, Montana,
Oregon, Washington)

Region XIV—Los Angeles
1340 West 6th Street
Los Angeles, California 90017
(213) 688-2650
(California, Hawaii, Nevada)

_____

There is no Region IX.

Index

About the Author

A. Michael Pascal is owner and president of United Bureau of Investigation, Inc., doing business out of Braintree, Massachusetts. He attended MIT and received a degree in criminology from Northeastern University. The author has provided extensive security programs not only for the medical facilities in the greater Boston area, but also for institutions and facilities in other parts of the country.

As president of the Massachusetts Associated Licensed Detective Agencies and a member of the World Association of Detectives, Mr. Pascal has participated throughout the world in seminars on security and investigation. He has also been instrumental in drafting legislation on behalf of the security profession and has served as a special investigator for the office of the Massachusetts Attorney General. Mr. Pascal is a member of the Massachusetts Chiefs of Police Association.